RENAL DIET COOKBOOK

200 Simple, Fast, and Nutritious Dishes for Chronic Kidney Disease Management

JADEN MALLIN

TABLE OF CONTENTS

Introduction

The kidneys' primary job is filtering and purifying the body's waste and surplus vital minerals and performing other tasks. The discovery of chronic renal illness will induce worry and alarm due to the essential function. Doctors and nutritionists have learned how to manage an essential component in preventing, postponing, or even stopping kidney disease: food. What you eat has a significant impact on the health of your kidneys. However, preparing meals that fulfil the requirements of a renal diet while still being easy and delicious may be difficult and time-consuming.

People with poor kidney function should follow a kidney or renal diet to decrease waste within their blood. Consumption of food and beverages is a source of waste within the blood. When the kidneys' function is impaired, they are unable to filter or remove waste effectively. If waste is accumulated in the blood, it may damage a patient's electrolyte balance. A renal diet may help to improve kidney function and postpone the development of full-blown kidney failure.

A renal diet is low in salt, phosphorus, and protein. In most instances, a renal diet stresses the need of consuming high-quality protein and limiting fluid consumption. Some individuals may also need to limit their potassium and calcium intake. Because each patient's body is unique, they must work with a renal dietitian to prepare a diet that is customized to their particular requirements. This Renal Diet Cookbook includes a meal for kidney-friendly eating, lifestyle changes to control and prevent kidney disease, and a variety of delicious recipes (such as exact amounts of calories, carbohydrates, protein, dietary fibers, sodium, fat, potassium, and phosphorus) and servings per recipe to help you eat your way to better health.

1

What Is Kidney Disease?

Kidney illness may affect your body's ability to cleanse and filter your blood, as well as control your blood pressure. It may also affect red blood cell production and vitamin D metabolism, crucial for bone health.

When you are born, you have two kidneys. They're on each side of your spine, just above your waist.

If your kidneys are impaired, waste products and fluid may accumulate in your body. Swelling, ankle sprains, weakness, nausea, and shortness of breath are all potential adverse effects. Without treatment, the damage may increase, and your kidneys could cease functioning correctly.

This is significant since it may jeopardize your life.

Kidney Disease and Its Causes

Acute kidney disease - causes

Acute renal failure happens when your kidneys cease functioning suddenly. The major reasons are insufficient blood supply to the kidneys, direct renal damage, and urine backlog in the kidneys.

Chronic kidney disease - causes

Chronic renal disease is a disorder in which your kidneys stop working correctly for longer than three months. It's conceivable that you won't notice any symptoms at first, but that's when its simplest to treat. Diabetes (types 1 and 2) and high blood pressure are the most common causes. High blood sugar levels may harm your kidneys over time. High blood pressure also affects your blood vessels, particularly those that feed your kidneys.

What Is a Renal Diet and Its Benefits?

A renal diet is low in salt, phosphorus, and protein. In most instances, a renal diet stresses the need of consuming high-quality protein and limiting fluid consumption. Some individuals may also need to limit their potassium and calcium intake.

This diet is intended to maintain your body's minerals, electrolytes, and fluid levels balanced if you have CKD or are on dialysis. Dialysis patients must follow this diet to avoid waste products accumulating in the body.

A renal diet may help to improve kidney function and postpone the development of full-blown kidney failure.

A renal diet is low in salt, phosphorus, and protein. In most instances, a renal diet stresses the need of consuming high-quality protein and limiting fluid consumption. Some individuals may also need to limit their potassium and calcium intake. Because each patient's body is unique, they must work with a renal dietician to prepare a diet that is customized to their particular requirements.

Best Foods for People with Kidney Disease

Fatty fish

Tuna, salmon, and other cold-water fatty fish rich in omega-3 fatty acids may be a beneficial addition to any diet.

Omega-3 fatty acids are not produced by the body and must be acquired via food. Fatty fish has a high concentration of healthy fats.

According to the National Kidney Foundation, omega-3 fats may lower blood pressure and decrease fat levels in the blood. Finding natural ways to decrease blood pressure, a risk factor for kidney disease may protect the kidneys.

Sweet potatoes

Sweet potatoes are similar to white potatoes, but their high fiber content may allow energy to be broken down more quickly, resulting in a smaller insulin spike. Sweet potatoes also include minerals and vitamins, such as potassium, that may help balance salt levels in the body and reduce the effect on the kidneys.

On the other hand, sweet potato is a high-potassium food. As a result, anybody with CKD or on dialysis may wish to cut down on their consumption.

Dark leafy greens

Kale, spinach, and chard are nutritious leafy greens rich in vitamins, fiber, and minerals. Several of them include antioxidants and other beneficial compounds.

These items, however, may not be suitable for those on a low-potassium diet or those on dialysis due to their high potassium content.

Berries

Blueberries, strawberries, and raspberries, for instance, are rich in vitamins, minerals, and antioxidant components. These may aid in the protection of the body's cells. Berries are likely to satisfy a sweet craving better than other sugary meals.

Apples

Pectin, a kind of fiber, is found in apples, making them a portion of healthy food. Pectin may help to reduce the number of kidney-damaging risk factors, including high cholesterol and blood sugar. Apples are also a fantastic method to keep your sweet appetite in check.

Cabbage

Cabbage is a green vegetable that may be beneficial to those who suffer from renal disease. It contains a range of useful compounds and vitamins while being low in salt and potassium.

Red bell peppers

Red bell peppers are low in minerals, such as potassium and sodium and contain helpful antioxidant compounds to protect cells from damage.

Garlic

Garlic is an excellent flavoring choice for those with CKD. It may improve the taste of other foods while decreasing the need for salt. Garlic also offers several health benefits.

Cauliflower

Cauliflower is a versatile vegetable that may help those with chronic renal disease (CKD). It may be used to replace rice, mashed potatoes, or even pizza crust when correctly cooked. Cauliflower also has a wide range of nutrients while being low in sodium, potassium, and phosphorus.

Arugula

Many greens are out of the question for those with CKD, but arugula is a good alternative. Although arugula has less potassium than other greens, it does include fiber and other minerals.

Olive oil

Olive oil may be a healthy cooking oil due to the kind of fat it contains. Olive oil is high in oleic acid, a polyunsaturated fatty acid that may help in inflammation reduction.

Egg whites

The yolks of eggs are rich in phosphorus, making them a basic protein. For individuals with CKD, egg whites may be utilized to make scrambled eggs or omelets.

Foods to Avoid or Limit

The kidneys filter blood, remove waste via urine, produce hormones, control minerals, and maintain fluid balance.

A variety of factors may cause kidney disease. The most prevalent are uncontrolled diabetes and high blood pressure.

Alcoholism, hepatitis C, heart disease, and HIV may all lead to kidney damage.

When the kidneys become damaged and unable to function properly, fluid may build up in the blood, and waste can collect in the circulation.

However, removing or limiting some items from your diet may help reduce waste product buildup in the blood, improve kidney function, and avoid further damage.

Dark-colored soda

Dark-colored sodas contain phosphorus-containing chemicals. Phosphorus is added to many foods and drinks throughout the production process to enhance taste, prolong shelf life, and prevent discoloration. Natural, animal-based, and plant-based phosphorus are absorbed more slowly by your body than this extra phosphorus.

In the form of tastes, phosphorus is not linked to protein-like natural phosphorus. Rather, it's generated in the same way as salt is, and the digestive tract easily absorbs it. Additive phosphorus is typically included in a product's ingredient list. On the other hand, food producers cannot list the precise amount of added phosphorus on the label. While the quantity of additive phosphorus in a 200-mL drink varies depending on the kind of soda, it is estimated that all dark-colored sodas contain 50–100 mg.

According to the United States Department of Agriculture's food database, a 12-ounce cola has 33.5 mg of phosphorus. Therefore, drinks, especially dark sodas, should be avoided on a renal diet.

Avocados

Avocados are renowned for their high fiber content, heart-healthy fats, and antioxidants, among other things.

Avocados are usually a nutritious complement to a meal, but individuals with renal disease should avoid them.

Avocados are a good source of potassium. As a result, they're an excellent source. Potassium is found in 690 milligrams in a single avocado of average size.

People with renal disease may still consume avocados if they limit their food intake to one-fourth of avocado and limit their potassium consumption.

Avocados, especially guacamole, should be restricted or avoided if you're on a renal diet and need to minimize your potassium intake. However, keep in mind that everyone's needs are different, and the most important factor to consider is your overall diet and health objectives.

Canned foods

Canned goods such as vegetables, soups, and beans are often bought due to their cheap cost and convenience.

On the other hand, most canned goods have a high sodium content due to salt as a preservative to prolong their shelf life.

Canned foods have a high salt content; therefore, those with renal disease are frequently recommended to avoid or restrict their consumption.

Furthermore, washing and draining canned goods like beans and tuna may decrease salt levels by 38–80 percent, depending on the product.

Whole wheat bread

Picking the right bread for individuals with renal disease may be challenging.

For healthy individuals, whole wheat bread is often recommended over refined white flour bread.

Whole-wheat bread may be a healthier choice due to its higher fiber content. However, white bread is favored over whole wheat bread by individuals with renal disease. This is due to its high phosphorus and potassium content. The more bran or whole grains a loaf of bread has, the greater its potassium and phosphorus levels. For example, a 1-ounce portion of whole wheat bread contains 57 mg of phosphorus and 69 mg of potassium. White bread, on the other hand, only contains 28 mg of phosphorus and potassium per serving.

Consuming one slice of whole wheat bread rather than two may help reduce your phosphorus and potassium consumption without eliminating whole wheat bread. It's essential to note that most bread and bread products have a high salt level, whether white or whole wheat. Compare the nutritional labels of several kinds of bread, choose a low-salt option if feasible, and keep note of your portion sizes.

Brown rice

Brown rice, as well as whole-wheat bread, is a whole grain that contains more phosphorus and potassium than white rice.

Cooked brown rice contains 150 mg of phosphorus and 154 mg of potassium per cup, compared to 54 mg of potassium and 69 mg of phosphorus in cooked white rice.

Brown rice may be used in a renal diet if portion sizes are controlled and balanced with other meals to avoid excessive daily potassium and phosphorus consumption. Low-phosphorus cereals such as bulgur, pearled barley, buckwheat, and couscous may be substituted for brown rice.

Bananas

Bananas are well-known for their potassium content.

While bananas are usually low in sodium, each medium banana has 422 mg of potassium.

If you've been advised to cut down on your potassium intake, eating a banana every day may be difficult. Several other tropical fruits, on the other hand, are rich in potassium. On the other hand, Pineapples contain less potassium than other tropical fruits, making them a healthier yet enjoyable option.

Dairy

Dairy products are high in vitamins and minerals. They're also a natural supply of phosphate and potassium and a good source of protein. For example, 1 cup (240 mL) whole milk has 349 mg of potassium and 222 mg of phosphorus. Excessive dairy intake, especially coupled with other phosphorus-rich meals, may be detrimental to bone health in individuals with renal disease. This may come as a surprise since milk and dairy products are often recommended for strong bones and muscles.

On the other hand, ingesting too much phosphorus may cause a buildup of phosphorus in the blood, which can deplete calcium levels if your kidneys are compromised. This may cause your bones to shrink and weaken over time, increasing your chance of breaking or fracture. Dairy products are similarly high in protein. 8 grammes of protein are found in a cup of whole milk (240 mL).

It may be essential to limit dairy intake to decrease protein waste in the blood. Unenriched almond milk and rice milk are dairy substitutes that are lower in phosphorus, potassium, and protein than cow's milk, making them ideal for those on a renal diet.

Oranges and orange juice

Orange juice and oranges are known for their high vitamin C content, but they also contain potassium. A big orange has 333 mg of potassium (184 grams). In addition, 1 cup of orange juice has 473 mg of potassium in it.

Due to their high potassium content, orange juice and oranges should be avoided or limited on a renal diet. Apples, grapes, cranberries, and liquids are good substitutes for orange juice and oranges since they contain less potassium.

Processed meats

Processed meats have long been associated with chronic illnesses, and their high preservative content is generally regarded as dangerous. Processed meats are those that have been salted, cured, dried, or canned. Just a few examples are hot dogs, pepperoni, bacon, jerky, and sausage. Processed meats include a lot of salt, which improves the taste and preserves the flavor.

Consequently, keeping your daily salt consumption below 2,300 mg may not be easy if you consume a lot of processed meat. In addition, processed meats are high in protein. If you've been told to limit your protein intake, it's also a good idea to limit your intake of processed meats.

Lifestyle Changes to Manage Chronic Kidney Disease

Certain lifestyle changes may help to delay the progression of chronic renal disease (CKD). These changes may also aid in the prevention of other disease-related health problems. Lifestyle changes may be required depending on the stage of CKD. They will also be influenced by any other health problems you may be experiencing. You may be asked to:

- _Maintain a Healthy Blood Pressure Level_

High blood pressure is a common cause of CKD. If you already have high blood pressure, you may need to change your diet. Medicines may be prescribed to help you maintain a normal blood pressure level.

- _Get Rid of Extra Weight_

Diabetes and high blood pressure may be caused by obesity or excess weight. Your doctor or a nutritionist can help you figure out how to lose weight safely.

- _Maintain a Healthy Blood Glucose Level_

High blood glucose levels aggravate CKD. You can tell whether you have diabetes by doing a few simple tests. You may need to change your diet if this is the case. Medicines may be prescribed to help you maintain a normal blood glucose level.

- _Quit Smoking_

CKD is exacerbated by smoking. Your doctor will explore a variety of alternatives for helping you effectively stopping smoking.

- _Alter Your Eating Habits_

When table salt and dietary protein are eaten, CKD develops more rapidly. Phosphorus, a mineral included in certain foods, remains in the blood when the kidneys aren't working correctly. Phosphorus may weaken bones as a result of calcium loss. CKD may also cause an increase in the number of lipids in your blood. As a consequence, a stroke or a heart attack may ensue.

Your doctor may place restrictions on salt, dairy products, protein, peas, cola, almonds, and high-fat meals. A dietitian can help you make healthier food choices. A dietician can help you make the most of what you eat if you have CKD and don't feel like eating.

- ***Exercise regularly***

You may achieve or maintain physical fitness with the help of an exercise training plan. This, in combination with other lifestyle changes, may help to lower the risk of coronary heart disease and depression. Both of these conditions are prevalent among CKD patients.

2

Smoothies Recipes

Homemade Flavored Coffee Creamer

INGREDIENTS:

- 1 can or 14 oz condensed milk, sweetened
- 2 c. milk

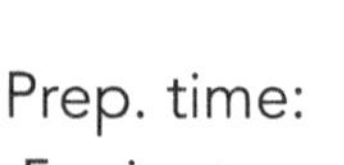

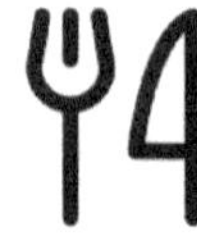

Prep. time:
5 minutes

Cooking time:
10 minutes

Servings:
15

NUTRITION PER SERVING:

- Calories: 83 Cal
- Protein: 2 g
- Carbs: 3 g
- Fat: 2 g

DIRECTIONS:

1. Shake a 32-ounce jar half full of condensed milk plus milk vigorously.

2. Stir in the seasonings and shake it up well.

Party Punch

INGREDIENTS:

- 1-liter ginger ale, diet
- 1/2 cup of liquid pineapple concentrate
- 1-pint sherbet, lime-flavored

Prep. time:
5 minutes

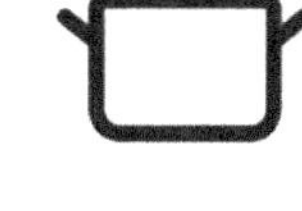

Cooking time:
10 minutes

Servings:
13

NUTRITION PER SERVING:

- Calories: 63 Cal
- Protein: 0 g
- Carbs: 4 g
- Fat: 1 g

DIRECTIONS:

1. Put the ginger ale to a dish or punch bowl and stir to combine.
2. After putting the pineapple concentrate, carefully combine everything.
3. Mix the sherbet with a scoop.
4. Serve when the sherbet begins to melt.

Atol de Maíz A Mexican Corn Drink

INGREDIENTS:

- 4 ears corn on the cob
- 4 cups almond milk or water
- 1 tsp. of vanilla extract
- Cinnamon sticks, optional for garnish
- 1 tsp. of cocoa powder
- 2 tbsps. of honey
- 1 tbsp. of cinnamon

NUTRITION PER SERVING:

- Calories: 65 Cal
- Protein: 2 g
- Carbs: 4 g
- Fat: 1.5 g

  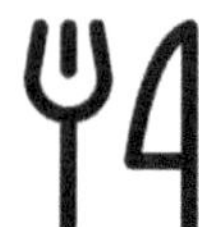

Prep. time:
10 minutes

Cooking time:
10 minutes

Servings:
4

DIRECTIONS:

1. Remove the kernels with a sharp knife to form 3 cups. Combine 2 1/2 cups maize and 2 cups water in a blender.

2. Drain the blended corn through a sieve in a saucepan. Combine the remaining maize kernels, one-third cup sugar, and 1 tsp. vanilla essence in a mixing bowl. If desired, 2 tbsp. honey with 1 tbsp. cinnamon or 1 tsp. chocolate powder may be added.

3. Bring to a boil over medium-high heat, then lower the heat and simmer for another 5 minutes, or until the sauce has thickened.

4. Serve immediately after pouring into a dish and sprinkling with cinnamon.

5. Put the cinnamon stick at the end if desired.

Watermelon Lime Refresher

INGREDIENTS:

- 2 limes
- 4 cups watermelon, cubed
- 2 cups strawberries
- 2 cups ice
- 6 large basil leaves

NUTRITION PER SERVING:

- Calories: 56 Cal
- Protein: 1 g
- Carbs: 14 g
- Fat: 0 g

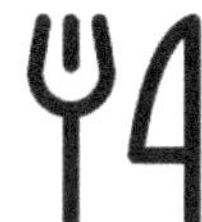

Prep. time:
5 minutes

Cooking time:
7 minutes

Servings:
6

DIRECTIONS:

1. Puree the lime juice, watermelon, and strawberries within a blender until smooth.

2. Finish with a layer of ice. Blend for around 30 secs to 1 minute, or until the mixture is completely smooth.

3. If desired, garnish with diced strawberries and basil leaves in separate glasses.

Watermelon Cooler

INGREDIENTS:

- 1 small grapefruit
- 2 cups cubed watermelon
- 8 ice cubes
- 1 1/2 cups water
- pinch of sea salt
- 1 tsp. of honey

 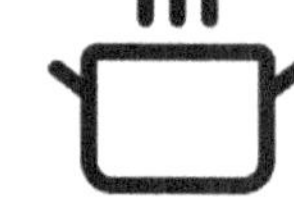

Prep. time:
5 minutes

Cooking time:
10 minutes

Servings:
3

NUTRITION PER SERVING:

- Calories: 59 Cal
- Protein: 1 g
- Carbs: 15 g
- Fat: 0 g

DIRECTIONS:

1. Remove the membrane from the grapefruit once it has been peeled. Sort the items into three groups.

2. Blend all the ingredients, except for the honey, within the blender until smooth.

3. Shake for the next 15 seconds after adding the honey. Serve as soon as possible. Enjoy!

Aromatic Tea

INGREDIENTS:

- 5 cups water
- 2 cinnamon sticks
- 1 (2-inch) piece ginger, peeled and sliced
- 1 (2-inch) piece turmeric, peeled and sliced
- 5 black peppercorns

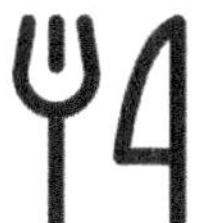

Prep. time:
20 minutes

Cooking time:
35 minutes

Servings:
5

NUTRITION PER SERVING:

- Calories: 0 Cal
- Protein: 0 g
- Carbs: 0 g
- Fat: 0 g

DIRECTIONS:

1. Fill the saucepan halfway with water and bring to a boil over medium heat.
2. Bring all the spices to a boil in a saucepan.
3. Reduce the heat to low and cook for an additional 30 minutes
4. Warm and cold serving temperatures are also acceptable. Enjoy!

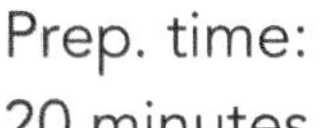

Mulled Apple Cider

INGREDIENTS:

- 4 cups of apple cider
- 2 sticks cinnamon
- 3 cloves
- 5 allspices
- 2 crushed cardamom pods

NUTRITION PER SERVING:

- Calories: 117 Cal
- Protein: < 1 g
- Carbs: 29 g
- Fat: < 1 g

Prep. time:
10 minutes

Cooking time:
15 minutes

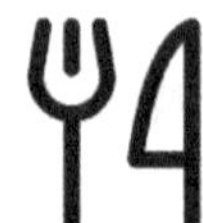

Servings:
4

DIRECTIONS:

1. Bring your cider to a low simmer within a medium-sized saucepan. Reduce the heat to a low setting and maintain it.

2. Mix in the spices well.

3. Simmer for around 10-15 minutes, occasionally stirring, allowing the spices to permeate the cider.

4. Enjoy it by pouring it into glasses.

Green Kiwi Smoothie

INGREDIENTS:

- 1 cup of water
- 1/2 avocado, peeled and chopped
- 1 kiwi, peeled and chopped
- 1/2 cup kale stemmed and chopped (fresh or frozen)
- 2 tbsp. almonds
- 2 ice cubes
- 1 tsp. of honey (optional)

NUTRITION PER SERVING:

- Calories: 99 Cal
- Protein: 2 g
- Carbs: 3 g
- Fat: 8 g

 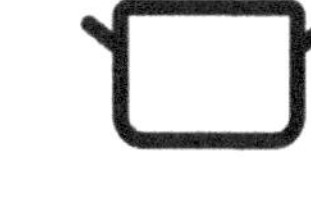 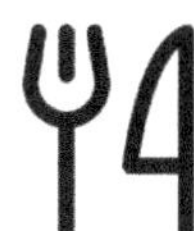

Prep. time: 10 minutes

Cooking time: 5 minutes

Servings: 2

DIRECTIONS:

1. Combine the kale, avocado, water, honey (optional), and kiwi in a blender. Blend until completely smooth and creamy.

2. Blend in the smashed ice until the mix is thick and creamy.

3. Pour the contents into separate glasses and serve immediately.

Pretty Pink Smoothie

INGREDIENTS:

- 1-liter ginger ale, diet
- 1/2 cup of liquid pineapple concentrate
- 1-pint sherbet, lime-flavored

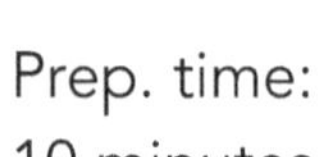

Prep. time: 10 minutes

Cooking time: 5 minutes

Servings: 2

NUTRITION PER SERVING:

- Calories: 146 Cal
- Protein: 2 g
- Carbs: 30 g
- Fat: 3 g

DIRECTIONS:

1. Blend the ginger, pear, rice milk, beet, flaxseed, and orange in a blender until smooth.

2. Combine the other ingredients in a blender and blend until smooth.

3. Blend in the smashed ice till the consistency is thick and smooth.

4. Pour the mixture into two big glasses and serve right away.

Homemade Rice Milk

INGREDIENTS:

- 1 cup white rice, cooked
- 4 cups water (filtered) and more for soaking

Prep. time:
10 minutes

Cooking time:
25 minutes

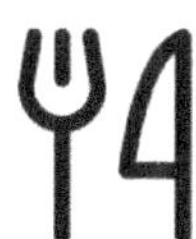

Servings:
1

NUTRITION PER SERVING:

- Calories: 112 Cal
- Protein: 0 g
- Carbs: 24 g
- Fat: 0 g

DIRECTIONS:

1. Pulse the water and rice in a food processor (or blender) for approximately 4 minutes or until smooth to make the rice creamy and smooth.

2. Pour the rice milk into a container after passing it through a fine sieve or folded cheesecloth. You may eliminate all liquid by squeezing the rice meal that has remained in the towel.

3. Remove the rice meal from the mixture and freeze the rice milk in an airtight glass jar for up to 1 week at room temp.

Strawberry Cheesecake Smoothie

INGREDIENTS:

- 1 cup rice milk, unsweetened
- 1 cup hulled strawberries
- 2 tbsps. cream cheese, at normal temperature
- 1/2 tsp. of honey
- 1 tsp. of vanilla extract
- 3-5 ice cubes

NUTRITION PER SERVING:

- Calories: 109 Cal
- Protein: 1 g
- Carbs: 13 g
- Fat: 6 g

Prep. time:
5 minutes

Cooking time:
5 minutes

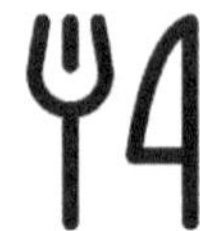

Servings:
2

DIRECTIONS:

1. Combine the strawberries, honey, ice cubes, vanilla, rice milk, and cream cheese in a blender and mix until smooth. In a food processor, puree until smooth, then serve.

2. In the cheesecake smoothie, replace the strawberries with your favorite fruit. Blackberries, raspberries, and blueberries are all excellent choices for this meal.

Cherry Citrus Mocktail

INGREDIENTS:

- 1/4 cup unsweetened tart cherry juice, unsweetened
- 1/2 cup or about 1 large fresh orange juice
- 1/4 cup or about 2 freshly squeezed lime juice
- 8-ozs soda can club
- 2 rings of lime or orange for garnish

NUTRITION PER SERVING:

- Calories: 55 Cal
- Protein: < 1 g
- Carbs: 14 g
- Fat: < 1 g

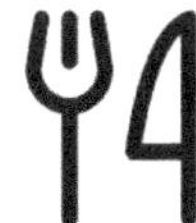

Prep. time:
5 minutes

Cooking time:
5 minutes

Servings:
2

DIRECTIONS:

1. In a glass container, combine all the juices.
2. Refrigerate after covering with a lid.
3. After taking the dish from the refrigerator, place it on a serving plate.
4. Fill a pair of colored cocktail glasses with the mixture. Finish with a splash of club soda.
5. On the rim of the glass, place an orange or lime slice.

Papaya Smoothie

INGREDIENTS:

- 3-ozs papaya, small pieces
- 1/2 cup almond or oat milk, unsweetened
- 1 tsp. of honey
- 1/2 tsp. ginger, fresh grated
- 2 tbsps. of lime juice
- 2 ice cubes

NUTRITION PER SERVING:

- Calories: 84 Cal
- Protein: 1 g
- Carbs: 18 g
- Fat: 2 g

  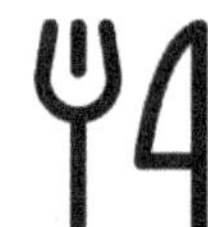

Prep. time: 5 minutes

Cooking time: 10 minutes

Servings: 1

DIRECTIONS:

1. In a blender, puree the lime, milk, ginger, papaya, and honey till smooth.
2. After that, process this for 15 secs at a medium speed.
3. Fill the container with ice cubes.
4. Blend 30 secs, or longer if required, at high speed to achieve smoothness; repeat if required.
5. Pour the mix into glasses and serve immediately.

Iced Tea with Orange and Mint

INGREDIENTS:

- 1/2 gallon water, boiling
- 4 black tea bags
- 2 oranges, large, washed and sliced
- 2 sprigs fresh mint leaves, large and washed

NUTRITION PER SERVING:

- Calories: 18 Cal
- Protein: < 1 g
- Carbs: 10 g
- Fat: 0 g

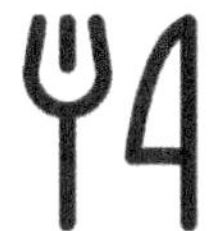

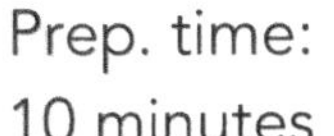

Prep. time:
10 minutes

Cooking time:
15 minutes

Servings:
8

DIRECTIONS:

1. In a mixing dish, combine the boiling hot water and tea bags. Allow 3 to 5 minutes for the tea to brew to your preferred strength.

2. Refrigerate it for 2 to 3 hours before serving.

3. After adding the orange pieces and mint, refrigerate the mixture for a few hours or overnight.

4. Serve on an ice bed.

Rose Hibiscus Limeade

INGREDIENTS:

- 8 cups of water
- 1/4 cup of maple syrup
- 2 pinches freshly grated ginger
- 1/3 cup dried hibiscus flowers
- 1/2 cup dried rose petals
- 2 limes, juiced

NUTRITION PER SERVING:

- Calories: 41 Cal
- Protein: 0 g
- Carbs: 11 g
- Fat: 0 g

Prep. time:
10 minutes

Cooking time:
25 minutes

Servings:
6

DIRECTIONS:

1. Over moderate flame, bring a stockpot 1/2 full of water to a boil.

2. When the water starts to boil, add the ginger and maple syrup to taste.

3. Reduce the heat to low and continue to cook for another 15 minutes

4. Combine the dried rose petals and dried hibiscus flowers with ginger-infused water in a large mixing bowl. Cook for a further 5 minutes

5. Strain the dried flower and grated ginger into a clean pitcher using a filter.

6. Lime juice and salt should be well combined in a large mixing bowl. The meal may be served chilled or at room temp.

Coco Coffee Frappe

INGREDIENTS:

- 8 cups of water
- 1/4 cup of maple syrup
- 2 pinches freshly grated ginger
- 1/3 cup dried hibiscus flowers
- 1/2 cup dried rose petals
- 2 limes, juiced

NUTRITION PER SERVING:

- Calories: 37 Cal
- Protein: < 1 g
- Carbs: 6 g
- Fat: 2 g

 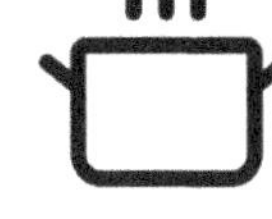

Prep. time:
10 minutes

Cooking time:
5 minutes

Servings:
2

DIRECTIONS:

1. Over moderate flame, bring a stockpot 1/2 full of water to a boil.

2. When the water starts to boil, add the ginger and maple syrup to taste.

3. Reduce the heat to low and continue to cook for another 15 minutes

4. Combine the dried rose petals and dried hibiscus flowers with ginger-infused water in a large mixing bowl. Cook for a further 5 minutes

5. Strain the dried flower and grated ginger into a clean pitcher using a filter.

6. Lime juice and salt should be well combined in a large mixing bowl. The meal may be served chilled or at room temp.

Cantaloupe Crush

INGREDIENTS:

- 1/2 cantaloupe
- 1 cup skim milk, fat-free
- 1 1/2 cup ice
- Sweetener to taste or about 1-2 tsps. sugar

NUTRITION PER SERVING:

- Calories: 50 Cal
- Protein: 3 g
- Carbs: 10 g
- Fat: 0 g

Prep. time:
5 minutes

Cooking time:
5 minutes

Servings:
4

DIRECTIONS:

1. Over moderate flame, bring a stockpot 1/2 full of water to a boil.
2. When the water starts to boil, add the ginger and maple syrup to taste.
3. Reduce the heat to low and continue to cook for another 15 minutes
4. Combine the dried rose petals and dried hibiscus flowers with ginger-infused water in a large mixing bowl. Cook for a further 5 minutes
5. Strain the dried flower and grated ginger into a clean pitcher using a filter.
6. Lime juice and salt should be well combined in a large mixing bowl. The meal may be served chilled or at room temp.

Lemonade

INGREDIENTS:

- Water, 2-1/2 cups

- Sugar, 1-1/4 cups
  (or sugar substitute)

- Lemon, finely shredded, 1/2 tsp.
  (or lime peel)

- Lemon, fresh, 1-1/4 cups
  (or lime juice)

- Ice cubes

NUTRITION PER SERVING:

- Calories: 108 Cal

- Protein: 0 g

- Carbs: 27 g

- Fat: 0 g

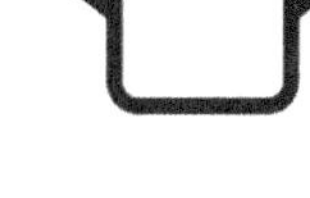

Prep. time:
5 minutes

Cooking time:
10 minutes

Servings:
6

DIRECTIONS:

1. In a medium saucepan, combine the water, sugar substitute or sugar and cook over medium heat until the sugar is dissolved. Remove from the heat and set aside to cool for around 20 minutes.

2. Toss the citrus juice and peel into the sugar mixture. Pour into a pitcher or container and cover to refrigerate. It may be stored in the refrigerator for up to three days.

3. In a glass packed with ice, combine 3 oz base and 3 oz water to prepare a glass of lemonade. Stir it up and eat it. You may freeze the remaining foundation in ice trays and use it as ice in beverages.

Watermelon Summer Cooler

INGREDIENTS:

- Crushed ice, 1 cup

- Seedless watermelon, 1 cup cubes

- Lime juice, 2 tsp.

- Sugar, 1 tbsp.

- Watermelon wedges, 2, small for garnish

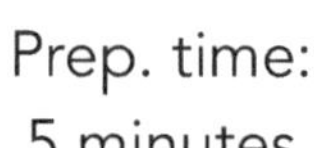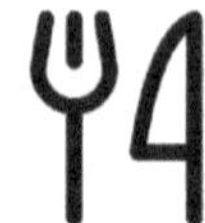

Prep. time:
5 minutes

Cooking time:
5 minutes

Servings:
2

DIRECTIONS:

1. Blend all the ingredients within your blender for around 30 secs, except the wedges separated for garnish.

2. Serve in two medium glasses garnished with lemon wedges.

NUTRITION PER SERVING:

- Calories: 52 Cal

- Protein: 0 g

- Carbs: 13 g

- Fat: 0 g

Four Ingredient Simple Blueberry Smoothie

INGREDIENTS:

- Frozen blueberries, 1/4 cup

- Rice milk, 1 cup

- Honey 1 tsp. (or stevia)

- Fresh mint, 1 sprig

- Ice cubes (to obtain desired thickness)

  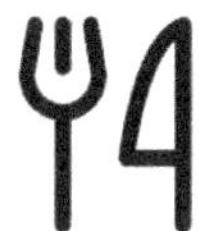

Prep. time:
5 minutes

Cooking time:
10 minutes

Servings:
1

DIRECTIONS:

1. In a blender, combine the blueberries, rice milk, honey, additional ice, and mint. Fill a large glass halfway with ice. Serve

NUTRITION PER SERVING:

- Calories: 70 Cal

- Protein: 0.3 g

- Carbs: 16.5 g

- Fat: 0.5 g

Kidney Nourishing Smoothie

INGREDIENTS:

- Cucumber, 1/2 large (peeled and sliced)
- Blueberries, fresh/frozen,1 cup
- Coconut water, 1 cup (or any nut milk or plain filtered water)
- Chia seeds or ground flax, 1-2 tbsp.
- Cinnamon, 1 pinch
- Lime juice, fresh, a good squeeze
- Ice, 1 cup
- Stevia (to taste), optional

 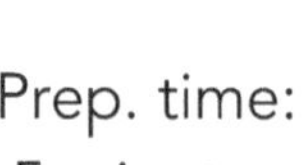  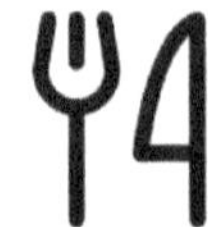

Prep. time:
5 minutes

Cooking time:
10 minutes

Servings:
7

DIRECTIONS:

1. Combine all the ingredients in a high-powered blender and seal the lid.
2. Start the machine and gradually raise the speed until it reaches the highest setting.
3. While processing, scrape the sides of the blender with a spatula as needed.
4. Blend for another 60-90 secs, or until the desired consistency is achieved.
5. Serve and have fun.

NUTRITION PER SERVING:

- Calories: 70 Cal
- Protein: 0.3 g
- Carbs: 16.5 g
- Fat: 0.5 g

Mixed Berry Protein Smoothie

INGREDIENTS:

- Cold water, 4 oz
- Mixed berries, fresh or frozen, 1 cup
- Ice cubes, 2
- Crystal light, 1 tsp., flavor enhancer drops (liquid, any berry flavor)
- Cream topping, 1/2 cup whipped
- Whey protein, 2 scoops of powder

  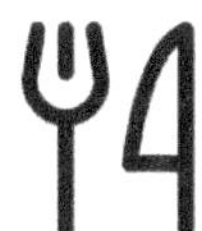

Prep. time:
10 minutes

Cooking time:
5 minutes

Servings:
7

DIRECTIONS:

1. In a blender, combine frozen berries, water, ice cubes, and crystal light drop. Blend until smooth and slushy.
2. Mix in the protein powder well.
3. Mix in the cream topping well.

NUTRITION PER SERVING:

- Calories: 152 Cal
- Protein: 14 g
- Carbs: 15 g
- Fat: 4 g

Easy Pineapple Protein Smoothie

INGREDIENTS:

- pineapple sherbet, 3/4 cup (or sorbet)

- whey protein powder, vanilla flavor, 1 scoop

- water, 1/2 cup

- ice cubes, 2, optional

Prep. time:
5 minutes

Cooking time:
5 minutes

Servings:
10

DIRECTIONS:

1. In a blender, combine the whey pineapple sherbet, protein powder, and water (plus ice cubes if preferred).

2. Blend for around 30-45 secs and serve right away.

NUTRITION PER SERVING:

- Calories: 268 Cal

- Protein: 18 g

- Carbs: 40 g

- Fat: 4 g

Blueberry Blast Smoothie

INGREDIENTS:

- frozen blueberries, 1 cup
- Splenda, 8 packets
- protein powder, 6 tbsp.
- ice cubes, 8
- apple juice, 14 oz (no added sugar)

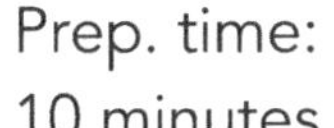

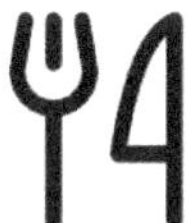

Prep. time:
10 minutes

Cooking time:
5 minutes

Servings:
4

DIRECTIONS:

1. Blend all the ingredients within your blender until smooth.

NUTRITION PER SERVING:

- Calories: 108 Cal
- Protein: 9 g
- Carbs: 18 g
- Fat: 0 g

What a Peach

INGREDIENTS:

- Raspberries, frozen, 1 cup
- Peach, 1 medium pit removed, sliced (or frozen peaches, 1/2 cup)
- Silken tofu, 1/2 cup
- Honey, 1 tbsp.
- Almond milk, vanilla flavored, unsweetened, 1 cup

 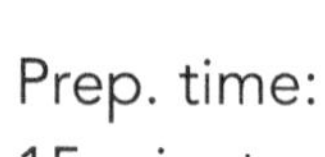  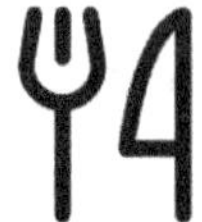

Prep. time:
15 minutes

Cooking time:
10 minutes

Servings:
2

DIRECTIONS:

1. In a blender, combine all ingredients and mix until smooth.

2. Fill a large glass halfway with ice.

NUTRITION PER SERVING:

- Calories: 70 Cal
- Protein: 0.3 g
- Carbs: 16.5 g
- Fat: 0.5 g

Very Berry Goodness

INGREDIENTS:

- Cucumber, 1 medium peeled and sliced
- Blueberries, fresh, 1/2 cup
- Strawberries, fresh or frozen, 1/2 cup
- Rice milk, 1/2 cup unsweetened
- Stevia to taste (optional)

  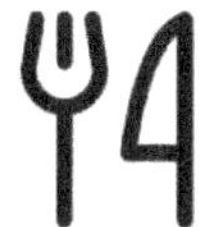

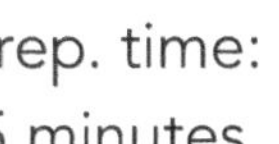

Prep. time:
5 minutes

Cooking time:
10 minutes

Servings:
1

DIRECTIONS:

1. In a blender, combine all your ingredients and mix until smooth.
2. Pour the cocktail into a large glass and serve.

NUTRITION PER SERVING:

- Calories: 152 Cal
- Protein: 14 g
- Carbs: 15 g
- Fat: 4 g

Bahama Breeze

INGREDIENTS:

- Strawberries, 1/2 cup
- Orange, 1 small, peeled
- Rice milk, 1/2 cup
- Handful of spinach
- Pineapple, 1/2 cup
- Ice cubes

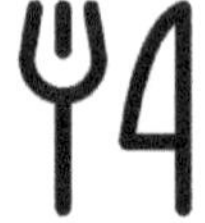

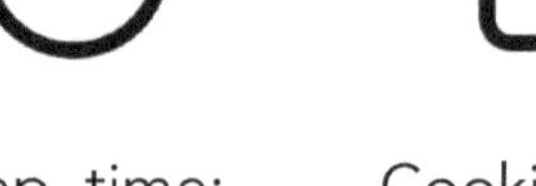

Prep. time:
15 minutes

Cooking time:
5 minutes

Servings:
1

DIRECTIONS:

1. Blend all the ingredients till smooth.
2. Serve immediately in a large glass.

NUTRITION PER SERVING:

- Calories: 108 Cal
- Protein: 0 g
- Carbs: 27 g
- Fat: 0 g

Cran-tastic

INGREDIENTS:

- Frozen cranberries, 1 cup
- Cucumber, 1 medium peeled and sliced
- Celery, 1 stalk
- Squeeze of lime
- A handful of parsley

   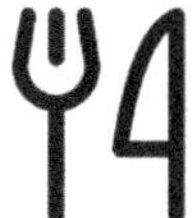

Prep. time:
10 minutes

Cooking time:
5 minutes

Servings:
1

DIRECTIONS:

1. In a blender, combine all the ingredients and mix until smooth.
2. Serve in a large glass.

NUTRITION PER SERVING:

- Calories: 70 Cal
- Protein: 0 g
- Carbs: 15 g
- Fat: 0 g

Watermelon Bliss

INGREDIENTS:

- Watermelon, 2 cups
- Cucumber, 1 medium, peeled and sliced
- Mint sprigs, 2, leaves only
- Celery stalk, 1
- Squeeze of lime
- Ice cubes

Prep. time:
5 minutes

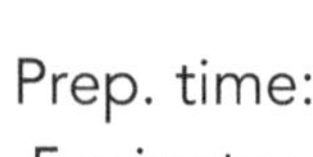

Cooking time:
10 minutes

Servings:
2

DIRECTIONS:

1. In a high-powered blender, combine all ingredients until completely smooth.
2. Pour the cocktail into a large glass, then serve.

NUTRITION PER SERVING:

- Calories: 52 Cal
- Protein: 0 g
- Carbs: 13 g
- Fat: 0 g

Chocolate Smoothie

INGREDIENTS:

- Whey protein, chocolate-flavored, 2 scoops
- Ice, 2 cups
- Southern comfort liqueur, 2 tbsp., (optional)
- Evaporated milk, 1/2 cup
- Condensed milk, 1/4 cup
- The ground cinnamon, 1/4 tsp.
- Nutmeg, pinch

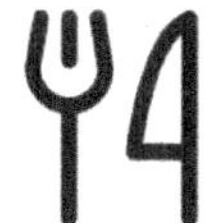
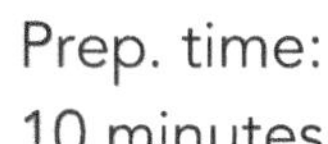

Prep. time:
10 minutes

Cooking time:
5 minutes

Servings:
4

DIRECTIONS:

1. Combine all your ingredients in your blender, except the cinnamon, and process on high for 1-2 minutes, or until smooth.

2. To serve, top with some whipped cream and a pinch of cinnamon.

NUTRITION PER SERVING:

- Calories: 142 Cal
- Protein: 10 g
- Carbs: 17 g
- Fat: 4 g

NOTES

3

Breakfast Recipes

Egg and Sausage Breakfast Sandwich

INGREDIENTS:

- Cooking spray (non-stick)
- 1/4 cup egg substitute, liquid
- Muffin 1 English
- Turkey sausage 1 patty
- Shredded cheddar cheese one tbsp.

NUTRITION PER SERVING:

- Calories: 188 Cal
- Protein: 4 g
- Carbs: 23 g
- Fat: 3 g

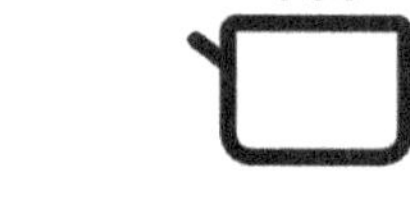

Prep. time:
15 minutes

Cooking time:
30 minutes

Servings:
1

DIRECTIONS:

1. Cook the egg mix over low heat in a small skillet sprayed with cooking spray. Flip the egg with a spatula when it's nearly done and cook for the next 30 secs.

2. Toasted English muffins are recommended.

3. Cover the turkey patty with a paper towel and microwave for 1 minute, until done as per the package instructions.

4. Make an English muffin with a fried egg on top. The other half of the muffin should be topped with a sausage patty, strong cheddar cheese, and the other half of the muffin.

Cowboy Caviar Bean and Rice Salad

INGREDIENTS:

- Corn 1/2 cup, cooked
- Rice 3 cups, cooked
- Lime juice 1/4 cup
- Canola oil 1/2 cup
- Brown sugar 2 tbsps.
- Dijon mustard 1 tbsp.
- Black pepper 1/2 tsp.
- Red bell pepper 1/2 cup, diced
- Black beans 1/2 cup, drained and rinsed
- Jalapeño 1, diced
- Cilantro 1/2 cup, chopped

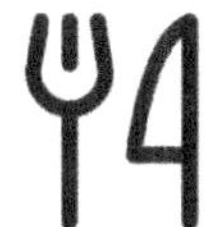
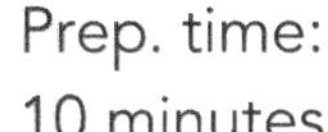

Prep. time: 10 minutes

Cooking time: 40 minutes

Servings: 6

DIRECTIONS:

1. Allow the rice and corn to cool before starting.
2. In a mixing bowl, whisk together the lime juice, brown sugar, oil, mustard, and black pepper to prepare the dressing.
3. In a large mixing bowl, combine all the remaining ingredients.
4. Toss the salad with the dressing to mix it.
5. Before serving, chill for one hr.

NUTRITION PER SERVING:

- Calories: 180 Cal
- Protein: 4 g
- Carbs: 20 g
- Fat: 2 g

Carrot Muffins

INGREDIENTS:

- 1/2 cup flour (all-purpose)
- Whole wheat flour 1/2 cup
- Oats 1/2 cup
- Ground flax seed 1/4 cup
- Baking powder 3/4 tsp.
- Baking soda 3/4 tsp.
- Cinnamon 3/4 tsp.
- Ginger 1/2 tsp.
- Brown sugar 1/2 cup
- Vegetable oil 1/2 cup
- Eggs 2 large
- 1/2 cup applesauce, unsweetened
- Fresh ginger, 2-inch piece
- Shredded carrots 2 cups

NUTRITION PER SERVING:

- Calories: 206 Cal
- Protein: 4 g
- Carbs: 12 g
- Fat: 12 g

Prep. time:
20 minutes

Cooking time:
25 minutes

Servings:
12

DIRECTIONS:

1. Preheat oven around 350°F.

2. Lightly coat muffin pans with nonstick spray.

3. Combine the dry ingredients in a large mixing bowl.

4. Combine wet ingredients in a medium mixing bowl using a whisk or fork.

5. Stir together the wet and dry ingredients until barely mixed.

6. Toss in some shredded carrots.

7. Fill muffin pans evenly with batter.

8. Preheat your oven to 350°F and bake for around 10 minutes

Chicken N' Orange Salad Sandwich

INGREDIENTS:

- Chopped cooked chicken 1 cup
- Celery 1/2 cup, diced
- Green pepper 1/2 cup, chopped
- Onion 1/4 cup, finely sliced
- Mandarin oranges 1 cup
- Mayonnaise 1/3 cup

NUTRITION PER SERVING:

- Calories: 162 Cal
- Protein: 12 g
- Carbs: 6 g
- Fat: 10 g

 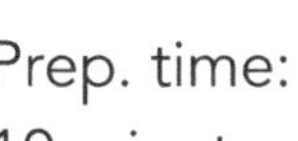  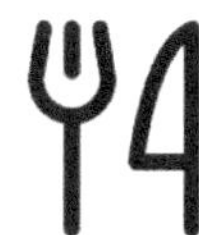

Prep. time:
10 minutes

Cooking time:
30 minutes

Servings:
6

DIRECTIONS:

1. Toss the celery, green pepper, chicken, and onion together.

2. In a mixing dish, combine the mandarin oranges and mayonnaise.

3. Gently combine the components.

4. With a piece of bread, serve.

Chinese Chicken Salad

INGREDIENTS:

- Ramen noodles 2 packages
- Olive oil 3 tbsps.
- Sesame seeds 2 tbsps.
- Chicken 2 cups
- Cabbage 1/2 head, shredded
- Green onions 4, diced
- Sugar 1/4 cup
- Sesame oil 1 tbsp.
- Rice vinegar 1/2 cup

NUTRITION PER SERVING:

- Calories: 203 Cal
- Protein: 19 g
- Carbs: 13 g
- Fat: 16 g

Prep. time: 10 minutes

Cooking time: 45 minutes

Servings: 8

DIRECTIONS:

1. Remove the ramen noodles from the package and crush them together.
2. Remove the seasoning packets from the packaging.
3. 1 tbsp. olive oil, warmed in a pan
4. In a mixing dish, combine dry noodles and sesame seeds.
5. On both sides, toast until golden brown.
6. In a large mixing bowl, combine the cabbage, turkey, or chicken, and green onions, then add the ramen noodles and sesame seeds.
7. Combine the sugar, 2 tbsps. olive oil, sesame oil, and vinegar.
8. Drizzle the dressing over the salad and toss to combine.

Cider Cream Chicken

INGREDIENTS:

- 4 chicken breasts, bone-in
- Unsalted butter 2 tbsps.
- Apple cider 3/4 cup

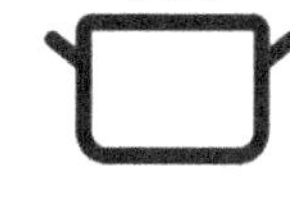
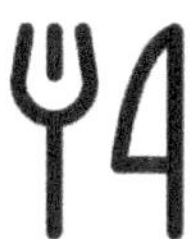

Prep. time:
15 minutes

Cooking time:
50 minutes

Servings:
8

NUTRITION PER SERVING:

- Calories: 186 Cal
- Protein: 27 g
- Carbs: 1 g
- Fat: 23 g

DIRECTIONS:

1. In a pan over medium-high heat, melt the butter. Both sides of the chicken should be browned.
2. Reduce the heat to medium-low and continue to cook for another 20 minutes
3. Take the chicken out of the pan.
4. Boiling the cider reduces it to about 1/4 cup.
5. Whisk in half-and-half over low heat until slightly thickened.
6. With a cream sauce, serve the chicken.

Chocolate-Orange Raisin Cookies

INGREDIENTS:

- 3 cups flour (all-purpose)
- 1 cup cocoa powder, unsweetened
- Baking powder 1 tbsp. low sodium
- Margarine 1 1/3 cups
- Powdered artificial sweetener 1/4 cup
- Eggs 4
- Orange juice 2/3 cup
- Raisins 2 cups

NUTRITION PER SERVING:

- Calories: 141 Cal
- Protein: 3 g
- Carbs: 17 g
- Fat: 1 g

 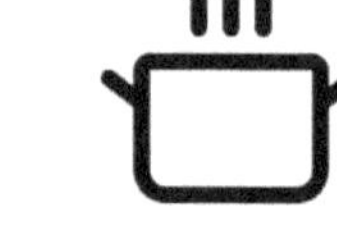

Prep. time:
25 minutes

Cooking time:
55 minutes

Servings:
36

DIRECTIONS:

1. Preheat oven around 375°F.

2. In a sifter, combine cocoa, flour, and baking powder.

3. With a stand/hand mixer, cream margarine until smooth, then add artificial sweetener.

4. Add the eggs and carefully beat them in.

5. Add the dry ingredients plus orange juice in that order.

6. Mix in the raisins well.

7. Drop teaspoonfuls of cookie dough onto baking sheets that haven't been buttered.

8. In the oven, bake for 10 minutes

9. Remove the baking sheet from the oven and put it aside to cool.

Coleslaw with a Kick

INGREDIENTS:

- Mayonnaise 1 cup
- Horseradish 1 tbsp.
- Cider vinegar 2 tsps.
- Granulated sugar 3 tbsps.
- Fresh dill 2 tsps., chopped
- Coleslaw mix with carrots, 1 lb.

NUTRITION PER SERVING:

- Calories: 107 Cal
- Protein: 0 g
- Carbs: 8 g
- Fat: 0 g

Prep. time:
25 minutes

Cooking time:
20 minutes

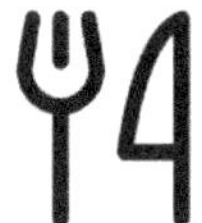

Servings:
10

DIRECTIONS:

1. In a large mixing bowl, combine the horseradish, mayonnaise, vinegar, sugar, and dill.

2. Stir in some coleslaw dressing until it's completely blended.

3. Chilling time should be at least one hr. It's best if you leave it in the fridge overnight.

Coleslaw with a Kick

INGREDIENTS:

- Bacon 12 slices
- Onions 2, chopped
- Chicken broth 7 cups, low sodium
- Potatoes 4
- Corn 8 cups
- Chicken breasts 8 boneless, diced
- Fresh thyme 6 tbsps., chopped
- Mocha Mix 4 cups
- Black pepper 1/2 tsp.
- Green onions 8, chopped

NUTRITION PER SERVING:

- Calories: 472 Cal
- Protein: 31 g
- Carbs: 55 g
- Fat: 6 g

Prep. time:
9 minutes

Cooking time:
15 minutes

Servings:
12

DIRECTIONS:

1. In a pan, cook bacon until crisp, then remove and set aside.

2. Sauté the onions in the bacon oil.

3. In a large saucepan, combine the potatoes and stock.

4. With the cover on, cook for 10 minutes

5. In a large mixing bowl, combine the chicken, corn and thyme.

6. Cook, covered until the chicken is cooked through (15 minutes).

7. Mocha must be stirred before serving. Cook for around 2 minutes after stirring into the liquid.

8. Mix in the pepper, bacon and green onions well.

Black-Eyed Peas

INGREDIENTS:

- Black-eyed peas 2 cups, dried
- Water 3½ cups
- Smoked turkey 12 ounces
- Onion 1 medium, finely chopped
- Garlic 6 cloves, finely chopped
- Celery 1 cup, diced
- Thyme 1/2 tsp.
- Ginger 1/2 tsp.
- Curry powder 1/2 tsp.
- Cayenne pepper 1 pinch

NUTRITION PER SERVING:

- Calories: 130 Cal
- Protein: 12 g
- Carbs: 19 g
- Fat: 9 g

  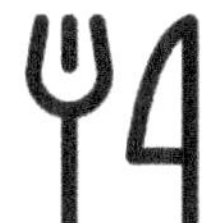

Prep. time: 10 minutes

Cooking time: 20 minutes

Servings: 12

DIRECTIONS:

1. Combine black-eyed peas and enough water to fill a large mixing bowl by 4 inches. Allow for at least six hours of soak time, ideally overnight.

2. Drain the peas and rinse them under cool water.

3. In a large saucepan, combine the black-eyed peas and the other ingredients.

4. Bring to a boil, then reduce to low heat, cover, and cook for around 1½ hours, or until peas are tender.

5. Once in a while, stir it.

Blasted Brussels sprouts

INGREDIENTS:

- Brussels Sprouts 2 cups
- Olive oil 2 tbsps.
- Parmesan Cheese 4 tbsps.
- Herb vinegar 1/4 cup

Prep. time:
5 minutes

Cooking time:
15 minutes

Servings:
4

NUTRITION PER SERVING:

- Calories: 68 Cal
- Protein: 3 g
- Carbs: 4 g
- Fat: 0 g

DIRECTIONS:

1. Preheat oven to around 450°F.

2. Get rid of any old leaves. Smaller sprouts must be left whole, whereas larger sprouts must be chopped in half.

3. Toss the sprouts with a little olive oil before starting.

4. Place the cookies on a lightly oiled baking sheet.

5. Cook for about 10 minutes Brussels sprouts are ripe when they are tender enough to be pierced with a fork.

6. Remove from the oven and top with fruit vinegar and freshly grated Parmesan cheese.

Broccoli Chicken Casserole

INGREDIENTS:

- Cooked broccoli 3 cups
- Onion 1 medium, chopped
- Chicken breast 3, diced
- Butter 2 tbsps.
- Eggs 2, beaten
- Milk 2 cups
- Cooked rice 2 cups
- Grated cheese 2 cups
- To top, grated parmesan

NUTRITION PER SERVING:

- Calories: 368 Cal
- Protein: 26 g
- Carbs: 26 g
- Fat: 22 g

Prep. time:
10 minutes

Cooking time:
1 hour 25 minutes

Servings:
6

DIRECTIONS:

1. Preheat oven around 350°F.

2. Microwave broccoli in a microwave-safe dish for 2-3 minutes, or until brilliant green, covered with plastic wrap.

3. In a separate pan, melt the butter and sauté the onion and chicken.

4. Bake all the ingredients in a buttered casserole dish.

5. Bake for 1 hour and 15 minutes, or until the middle is firm and a fork inserted in the center comes out clean.

Brown Bag Popcorn

INGREDIENTS:

- Popcorn kernels 1/4 cup
- Canola oil 1 tsp.
- 1 lunch bag (brown paper)

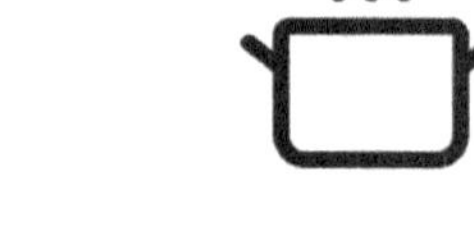

Prep. time:
5 minutes

Cooking time:
15 minutes

Servings:
1

NUTRITION PER SERVING:

- Calories: 155 Cal
- Protein: 4 g
- Carbs: 27 g
- Fat: 2 g

DIRECTIONS:

1. In a small mixing dish, combine the oil and popcorn.

2. Half-fill a brown bag with popcorn, fold it closed and staple the top twice.

3. Microwave for 3 minutes on medium, or until each pop lasts 5 seconds.

Burritos Rapides

INGREDIENTS:

- Olive oil 1 1/2 tsps.
- Red bell pepper 1/2, diced
- Green onions 4, sliced thin
- Eggs 8, beaten
- Corn tortillas 4

NUTRITION PER SERVING:

- Calories: 232 Cal
- Protein: 14 g
- Carbs: 16 g
- Fat: 10 g

 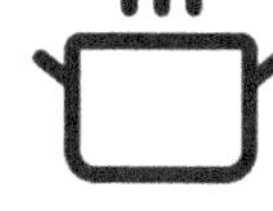 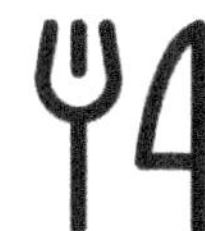

Prep. time:
8 minutes

Cooking time:
20 minutes

Servings:
4

DIRECTIONS:

1. Heat the oil in a large frying pan over medium heat.
2. Cook for around 3 minutes, or until the bell pepper and green onion have softened.
3. Scramble the eggs for around 5 minutes, or until they are fully cooked.
4. Place the tortillas between two wet paper towels on a platter.
5. Microwave the tortillas for around 2 minutes once they have been toasted.
6. Fill the tortillas with the egg mix while they are still heated.
7. Roll up the tortillas and eat them.

Beet Salad

INGREDIENTS:

- Beets 4, diced
- Walnuts 1/2 cup
- Leaf lettuce 1
- Fresh basil 1/4 cup, chopped fine
- Herb vinegar 1/2 cup
- Olive oil 2 tbsps.
- Blue cheese 3 ounces

NUTRITION PER SERVING:

- Calories: 283 Cal
- Protein: 6 g
- Carbs: 16 g
- Fat: 4 g

Prep. time:
10 minutes

Cooking time:
15 minutes

Servings:
4

DIRECTIONS:

1. Preheat your oven to around 400°F.
2. Beets should be roasted for 45 minutes or until soft.
3. Before peeling and dicing, let it cool.
4. Combine the sugar, almonds, and water in a frying pan. Heat the mixture, constantly stirring, until the liquid has almost evaporated.
5. Pour the nuts onto parchment paper and separate them while they are still hot after they are uniformly covered, and the frying pan is almost dry.
6. Allow for chilling before keeping at room temperature for many months.
7. Make a lettuce bed.
8. Toss the beets with the vinegar, basil, and oil in a mixing bowl.
9. Toss the lettuce into a bed.
10. On top, arrange the cheese cubes and almonds.

Banana-Apple

INGREDIENTS:

- Banana 1/2, peeled
- Plain yogurt 1/2 cup
- 1/2 cup applesauce (unsweetened)
- Skim milk 1/4 cup
- Honey 1 tbsp.
- Oat bran 2 tbsps.

NUTRITION PER SERVING:

- Calories: 292 Cal
- Protein: 9 g
- Carbs: 61 g
- Fat: 7 g

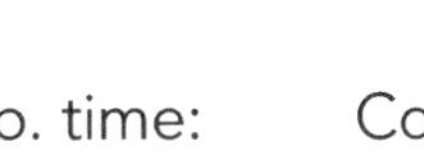

Prep. time:
5 minutes

Cooking time:
5 minutes

Servings:
1

DIRECTIONS:

1. Combine the banana, applesauce, yoghurt, milk, and honey in a blender.
2. Blend until the mixture is smooth.
3. Blend in the oat bran until it reaches a thick consistency.

Baked Potato Soup

INGREDIENTS:

- Potatoes 2 large
- Flour 1/3 cup
- Skim milk 4 cups
- Pepper 1/2 tsp.
- Monterey jack cheese 4 ounces
- 1/2 cup sour cream (fat-free)

NUTRITION PER SERVING:

- Calories: 216 Cal
- Protein: 15 g
- Carbs: 29 g
- Fat: 1 g

  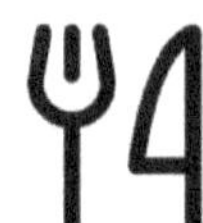

Prep. time:
18 minutes

Cooking time:
20 minutes

Servings:
6

DIRECTIONS:

1. Preheat the oven to around 400°F and bake the potatoes until they are fork soft.

2. Allow time for chilling.

3. By cutting lengthwise, scoop out the pulp.

4. Add the flour to a big pot. Gradually pour in the milk, stirring continuously until everything is well mixed.

5. Season with salt and pepper and toss in the potato pulp.

6. Cook, stirring continuously, over medium-high heat until the sauce is thick and boiling.

7. Add the cheese and stir until it melts.

8. Remove the skillet from the heat and stir in the sour cream.

Asian Pear Salad

INGREDIENTS:

- Sugar 1/2 cup
- Water 1/2 cup
- Walnuts 1/2 cup
- Green leaf lettuce 6 cups
- Asian pears 4
- Blue cheese 2 ounces
- Pomegranate seeds 1/2 cup
- Vinegar dressing

NUTRITION PER SERVING:

- Calories: 301 Cal
- Protein: 6 g
- Carbs: 41 g
- Fat: 1 g

Prep. time:
10 minutes

Cooking time:
35 minutes

Servings:
4

DIRECTIONS:

1. In a nonstick fry pan, dissolve the sugar and water.
2. Heat until you get a syrupy consistency.
3. Stir in the nuts quickly.
4. While the nuts are still hot, turn them out onto parchment paper and separate them. Allow cooling.
5. In a large mixing bowl, place the lettuce.
6. Toss lettuce with cheese, pears, and pomegranate seeds.
7. Serve with a nut topping and a vinegar dressing.

Apple Rice Salad

INGREDIENTS:

- Balsamic vinegar 2 tbsps.
- Olive oil 1 tbsp.
- Honey 2 tsps.
- Dijon mustard 2 tsps.
- Orange peel 1 tbsp.
- Garlic powder 1/4 tsp.
- Cooked rice 2 cups
- Apples 2 cups, chopped
- Celery 1 cup, thinly sliced
- 2 tbsps. sunflower seeds (unsalted)

NUTRITION PER SERVING:

- Calories: 238 Cal
- Protein: 4 g
- Carbs: 42 g
- Fat: 6 g

 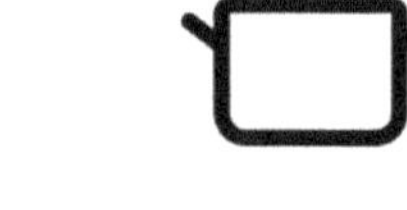

Prep. time: 10 minutes

Cooking time: 30 minutes

Servings: 4

DIRECTIONS:

1. Whisk together the olive oil, vinegar, honey, orange peel, mustard, and garlic powder after fully mixing, set aside.

2. In a large mixing bowl, combine the rice, celery, apples, and sunflower seeds. Toss until all the ingredients are equally distributed.

3. Toss the rice salad mix with the dressing until all the ingredients are well covered.

4. Serve immediately or refrigerate for up to 24 hours

Apple Bran Muffins

INGREDIENTS:

- Whole wheat flour 2 cups
- Wheat bran 1 1/2 cups
- Baking soda 1 1/4 tsps.
- Nutmeg 1/2 tsp.
- Orange rind 1 tbsp.
- Chopped apple 1 cup
- Raisins 1/2 cup
- 1/2 cup nuts, chopped
- Orange juice, 1
- Buttermilk 2 cups
- Egg 1 beaten
- Molasses 1/2 cup
- Oil 2 tbsps.

NUTRITION PER SERVING:

- Calories: 234 Cal
- Protein: 7 g
- Carbs: 40 g
- Fat: 8 g

Prep. time:
10 minutes

Cooking time:
30 minutes

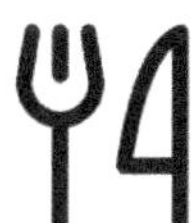

Servings:
3

DIRECTIONS:

1. Preheat oven to 350°F.

2. Using a fork, mix the flour, baking soda, bran, and nutmeg.

3. Toss together the orange peel, raisins, apples, almonds, and seeds in a mixing bowl.

4. Pour 1 cup orange juice into a 2-cup measuring cup, then add buttermilk to prepare 2 cups.

5. Combine the buttermilk, molasses, egg, and oil in a large mixing bowl and whisk until smooth.

6. Combine liquid and dry ingredients quickly with a few strokes.

7. Bake for around 30 minutes, filling muffin pans two-thirds full.

Acorn Squash Baked with Pineapple

INGREDIENTS:

- Acorn squash 1, seeded
- Unsalted butter (3 tbsps.)
- Brown sugar 2 tsps.
- Pineapple 3 tbsps., crushed
- Nutmeg 1/4 tsp.

NUTRITION PER SERVING:

- Calories: 202 Cal
- Protein: 2 g
- Carbs: 31 g
- Fat: 9 g

Prep. time:
10 minutes

Cooking time:
30 minutes

Servings:
4

DIRECTIONS:

1. Preheat oven to 400°F.

2. Place the squash cut side up on a baking sheet that has been prepped.

3. Put one tsp. butter and one tsp. brown sugar in each acorn half.

4. Wrap the squash in Al foil and bake until soft, about 30 minutes

5. Scoop cooked squash out of their shells, leaving a 1/4-inch-thick shell behind.

6. In a large mixing dish, combine cooked squash, 1 tbsp. butter, pineapple, and nutmeg. Blend until the mixture is smooth.

7. Fill shells halfway with the mixture and bake at 425°F for 15 minutes

Loaded veggie eggs

INGREDIENTS:

- Eggs 4 whole
- Cauliflower 1 cup
- 3 cups spinach, fresh
- Minced Garlic 1 clove
- Bell pepper 1/4 cup, chopped
- Onion 1/4 cup, chopped
- Black pepper 1/4 tsp.
- Oil of choice, 1 tbsp.
- Parsley, for garnish

NUTRITION PER SERVING:

- Calories: 240 Cal
- Protein: 15.3 g
- Carb: 8 g
- Fat: 16.6 g

Prep. time:
5 minutes

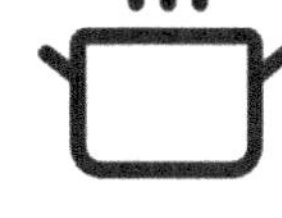

Cooking time:
7 minutes

Servings:
2

DIRECTIONS:

1. Set aside eggs that have been whisked till light and fluffy with pepper.

2. Heat the oil in a large skillet over medium heat.

3. Sauté the onions and peppers in a pan until the peppers are translucent and golden.

4. Before adding the cauliflower and spinach, rapidly whisk in the garlic.

5. After sautéing the veggies, cook for 5 minutes on medium-low heat.

6. Mix in the eggs with the veggies using a whisk.

7. Once the eggs are completely cooked, garnish with spring onions.

Spicy Tofu Scrambler

INGREDIENTS:

- Olive oil 1 tsp.
- Red bell pepper 1/4 cup, chopped
- Green bell pepper 1/4 cup, chopped
- Firm tofu 1 cup
- Onion powder 1 tsp.
- Garlic powder 1/4 tsp.
- Garlic 1 clove, minced
- Turmeric 1/8 tsp.

NUTRITION PER SERVING:

- Calories: 213 Cal
- Protein: 18 g
- Carbs: 10 g
- Fat: 13 g

 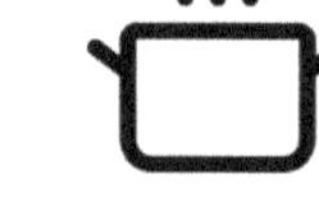

Prep. time:
10 minutes

Cooking time:
15 minutes

Servings:
2

DIRECTIONS:

1. In a medium-sized nonstick pan, sauté both bell peppers and garlic in olive oil.

2. Before breaking the tofu into the pan, it should be washed and drained. Stir in the remaining ingredients well.

3. Cook, stirring periodically, for approximately 20 minutes, or until the tofu becomes a little golden color. The mixture's water will evaporate.

4. A heated tofu scrambler is recommended.

Southwest Baked Egg Breakfast Cups

INGREDIENTS:

- Rice 3 cups, cooked
- Cheddar cheese 4 ounces, shredded
- Green chillies 4 ounces, diced
- Pimentos 2 ounces, diced and drained
- Skim milk 1/2 cup
- Eggs 2, beaten
- Ground cumin 1/2 tsp.
- Black pepper 1/2 tsp.
- Cooking spray (nonstick)

NUTRITION PER SERVING:

- Calories: 109 Cal
- Protein: 5 g
- Carbs: 13 g
- Fat: 4 g

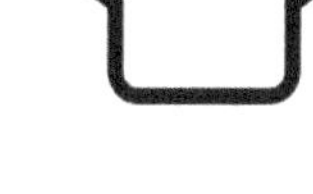

Prep. time:
5 minutes

Cooking time:
20 minutes

Servings:
12

DIRECTIONS:

1. Combine the rice, chiles, cheese, pimentos, eggs, milk, cumin, and pepper in a large mixing bowl.

2. Coat muffin cups with nonstick cooking spray.

3. Fill 12 muffin cups with the mixture equally. Sprinkle the remaining 2 ounces of cheese on top of each cup.

4. Preheat the oven to 400°F and bake for 15 minutes, or until golden brown.

Southwest Baked Egg Breakfast Cups

INGREDIENTS:

- Ground turkey 1 pound
- 8 burrito shells (6-inch)
- Canola oil 1/4 cup
- Eggs 8 beaten, scrambled
- Diced onions 1/4 cup
- 1/4 cup peppers, fresh bell
- 2 tbsps. jalapeño peppers, seeded
- 2 tbsps. scallions, fresh and chopped
- Cilantro 2 tbsps., chopped
- Chili powder 1/2 tsp.
- Smoked paprika 1/2 tsp.
- 1 cup Monterey Jack, shredded

  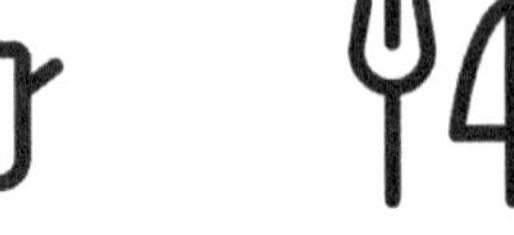

Prep. time:
25 minutes

Cooking time:
25 minutes

Servings:
8

DIRECTIONS:

1. Sauté the onions, scallions, meatloaf, peppers, and cilantro in half the oil until translucent. Remove the pan from the heat after adding the spices.

2. In a separate large sauté pan, heat the remaining oil and beaten eggs over medium-high heat.

3. Fill burrito shells halfway with vegetable and meatloaf mixture, cheese, eggs, then fold and serve.

NUTRITION PER SERVING:

- Calories: 407 Cal
- Protein: 25 g
- Carbs: 23 g
- Fat: 24 g

Apple and Zucchini Harvest Muffins

INGREDIENTS:

- Whole wheat pastry flour, 1 cup (or all-purpose flour if unavailable)
- All-purpose flour, 1/2 cup
- Ground flax seeds, 1/4 cup
- Baking powder, one tsp.
- Baking soda, 1/2 tsp.
- The ground cinnamon, 1 tsp.
- Canola oil, 1/3 cup
- Sugar, 1/4 cup
- Apple cider vinegar, 1 tbsp.
- Egg, 1
- Unsweetened applesauce, 1/2 cup
- Molasses, 1 tbsp.
- Zucchini, grated, 1 medium (about 1 cup)
- Shredded apple, 1/2 cup

NUTRITION PER SERVING:

- Calories: 178 Cal
- Protein: 3 g
- Carbs: 25 g
- Fat: 8 g

Prep. time:
10 minutes

Cooking time:
30 minutes

Servings:
12

DIRECTIONS:

1. Preheat the oven to 425°F.

2. For baking, coat a muffin pan with nonstick spray. Combine the flour, cinnamon, baking soda, flax seeds, and baking powder in a large mixing bowl.

3. Whisk the oil, apple cider vinegar, sugar, egg, molasses, and applesauce in a separate container until thoroughly combined. Combine the apples and zucchini in a mixing bowl.

4. Combine the dry ingredients first, then add the liquid components. A few times, stir to combine. Pour the batter into the muffin cups that have been prepared.

5. Cook for 5 minutes at 425°F before lowering the temperature to 350°F.

6. Warm the dish before serving.

Kale and Cheddar Frittata

INGREDIENTS:

- Large eggs, 8
- Olive oil, 2 tbsp.
- Lacinato kale, 4 oz. (about 1/2 bunch), tough stems removed and cut into ribbons
- Kosher salt, 1/4 tsp.
- Ground black pepper, 1/4 tsp.
- Red pepper flakes, 1/4 tsp. crushed
- Garlic, 2 cloves, minced
- English cheddar, 1 oz, shredded (or any sharp cheese)

NUTRITION PER SERVING:

- Calories: 248 Cal
- Protein: 16 g
- Carbs: 4 g
- Fat: 20 g

 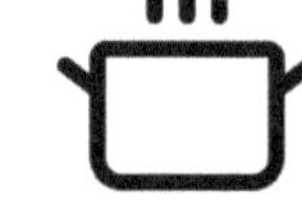

Prep. time: 10 minutes

Cooking time: 25 minutes

Servings: 4

DIRECTIONS:

1. Preheat the oven to 350°F.

2. In a separate dish, whisk together the eggs and set them aside.

3. Heat the oil in an oven-safe skillet over medium heat. Heat the kale, black pepper, salt, and red pepper until the kale begins to droop, stirring periodically. Add the garlic and continue to cook for another 2 minutes Remove the heat source.

4. Pour the beaten eggs into the heated skillet with the greens and stir to combine. Scatter the cheese on top and bake for approximately 10 minutes, or until the eggs are set. Cut each wedge into four equal pieces and serve.

Corn Pudding

INGREDIENTS:

- Kernel corn, 2 cups fresh cut or canned
- Eggs, 3 slightly beaten or egg substitute, 3/4 cup
- 1% milk, 1/2 cup
- Onion, 1/3 cup, finely chopped
- Water, 1/2 cup
- Butter, 1 tbsp., melted
- Granulated sugar, 1 tsp.
- Black pepper or white, 1 tsp.

NUTRITION PER SERVING:

- Calories: 120 Cal
- Protein: 6 g
- Carbs: 17 g
- Fat: 5 g

Prep. time:
15 minutes

Cooking time:
20 minutes

Servings:
6

DIRECTIONS:

1. Preheat your oven to 350°F.

2. In a mixing dish, combine all the ingredients.

3. Pour the mixture into a 12-quart casserole dish that has been oiled.

4. In a low pan filled with 1 inch of boiling water, place the casserole dish.

5. Bake for 40-45 minutes, or until the middle is set and a knife inserted in the center comes out clean.

6. Allow 10 minutes for it to come to room temp before serving.

French Toast

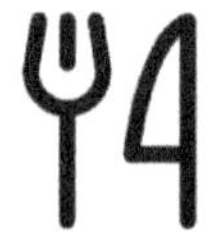

Prep. time:
10 minutes

Cooking time:
20 minutes

Servings:
4

INGREDIENTS:

- Egg whites, 4 large, slightly beaten
- 1% milk, 1/4 cup
- Cinnamon, 1/2 tsp.
- Allspice, 1/4 tsp.
- White bread, 4 slices (maybe toasted)
- Margarine, 1 tbsp.

NUTRITION PER SERVING:

- Calories: 125 Cal
- Protein: 7 g
- Carbs: 14 g
- Fat: 5 g

DIRECTIONS:

1. To the egg whites, add Combine the milk, allspice, and cinnamon in a mixing bowl.
2. At a time, one slice at a time, Bread should be dipped into the batter.
3. Melt margarine in a hot skillet. On the skillet, place a piece of bread.
4. Fry the bread till golden brown on both sides.
5. Drizzle with maple syrup and serve immediately (sugar-free if diabetic).

Creamy Pasta Salad

INGREDIENTS:

- Medium shells pasta 8 ounces
- Sour cream 1/2 cup
- Mayonnaise 1/2 cup
- Celery seed 1/2 tsp.
- Onion powders 1 tsp.
- Ground mustard 1/8 tsp.
- pickles 1/4 cup, chopped
- Celery 1 stalk, chopped
- Carrot 2 tbsps., grated

NUTRITION PER SERVING:

- Calories: 188 Cal
- Protein: 4 g
- Carbs: 23 g
- Fat: 2 g

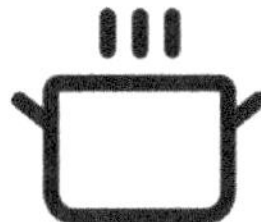
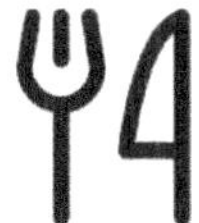

Prep. time:
10 minutes

Cooking time:
12 minutes

Servings:
8

DIRECTIONS:

1. After boiling the pasta according to the package instructions and washing it with cold water, set it aside.

2. Mix sour cream, celery seed, mayonnaise dressing, onion powder, and ground mustard.

3. Combine the cooked pasta and the dressing in a large mixing bowl.

4. Mix in the chopped pickles well.

5. As a garnish, add celery and carrots.

NOTES

4

Lunch Recipes

Acai Berry Smoothie Bowl

INGREDIENTS:

- 1 packet of frozen acai
- 1 cup of frozen berries mixed
- 3/4 cup of plain Greek yogurt (low fat)
- 1 tsp. of chia seeds
- 1/2 cup of rice milk
- 2 tbsps. of raspberries
- 2 tbsps. of blueberries
- 1/4 pear (fresh)

NUTRITION PER SERVING:

- Calories: 192 Cal
- Protein: 16 g
- Carbs: 28 g
- Fat: 4 g

Prep. time:
10 minutes

Cooking time:
30 minutes

Servings:
4

DIRECTIONS:

1. Shred whatever frozen acai puree you have.

2. Mix the acai, rice milk, Greek yoghurt, chia seeds, and mixed berries (frozen) in a blender.

3. Blend the ingredients until they are completely smooth. You should be able to consume it with a spoon if it has a thick enough consistency.

4. Divide the combined mix equally between two bowls.

5. Raspberry, blueberry, and sliced pear are served on top.

Egg and Sausage Sandwich

INGREDIENTS:

- 1 cooking spray nonstick
- 1/4 cup of low-cholesterol liquid
- 1 muffin (English)
- 1 sausage of a turkey patty
- 1 tbsp. of cheddar cheese (shredded)

NUTRITION PER SERVING:

- Calories: 253 Cal
- Protein: 17 g
- Carbs: 26 g
- Fat: 9 g

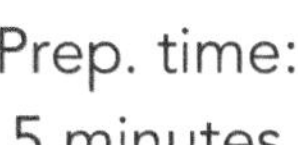

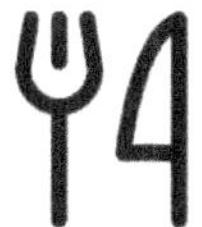

Prep. time:
5 minutes

Cooking time:
10 minutes

Servings:
2

DIRECTIONS:

1. Cook on low heat, pouring the egg mixture into a small pan coated with nonstick cooking spray. When the egg is nearly done, flip it with a spatula and cook for another 30 seconds.

Toast English muffin

1. In a microwave-safe dish, place a turkey sausage patty, cover with a paper towel, and heat for 1 minute or until done.

2. Assemble an English muffin with the cooked egg inside. Top with a sausage patty, cheddar cheese, and a half of a muffin.

Microwave Coffee Cup Egg Scramble

INGREDIENTS:

- 1 egg (large)
- 2 egg whites large
- 2 tbsps. of milk (low fat)
- 1/8 tsp. of black pepper

NUTRITION PER SERVING:

- Calories: 130 Cal
- Protein: 15 g
- Carbs: 11 g
- Fat: 8 g

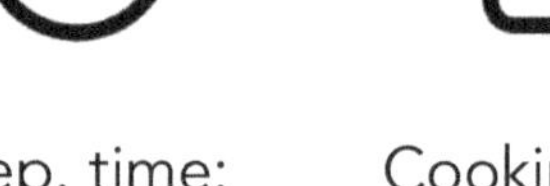

Prep. time:
5 minutes

Cooking time:
10 minutes

Servings:
1

DIRECTIONS:

1. Spray a 12-ounce coffee cup with nonstick cooking spray. In a cup, whisk together the milk, egg, and egg whites until smooth.

2. Cook for 45 seconds in a microwave-safe coffee cup; remove and stir. Cook in the microwave for another 30-45 seconds, or until the eggs are almost set.

3. Serve with a pinch of black pepper.

Quick and Easy Apple Oatmeal Custard

INGREDIENTS:

- 1/2, apple medium
- 1/3 cups of quick oatmeal cooking
- 1 egg large
- 1/2 cup of almond milk
- 1/4 tsp. of cinnamon

NUTRITION PER SERVING:

- Calories: 248 Cal
- Protein: 11 g
- Carbs: 33 g
- Fat: 8 g

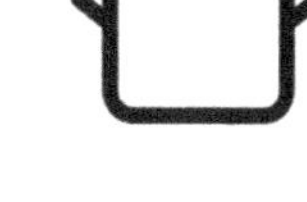

Prep. time:
10 minutes

Cooking time:
25 minutes

Servings:
4

DIRECTIONS:

1. 1/2 an apple, cored and coarsely sliced

2. In a large mixing bowl, combine the oats, egg, and almond milk. With a fork, thoroughly combine the ingredients. In a mixing dish, combine the apple and cinnamon. Stirring again until all the ingredients are well combined.

3. Cook for about 2 minutes on high in the microwave. With a fork, fluff the mixture. If necessary, cook for the next 30-60 seconds.

4. If you prefer a thinner porridge, add a bit of extra milk or even water.

Great Bagel

INGREDIENTS:

- 1 bagel of 2 oz.
- 2 tbsps. cream cheese
- 2 tomato slices, 1/4-inch thick
- 2 red onion slices
- 1 tsp. low-sodium lemon pepper seasoning

NUTRITION PER SERVING:

- Calories: 134 Cal
- Protein: 5 g
- Carbs: 19 g
- Fat: 6 g

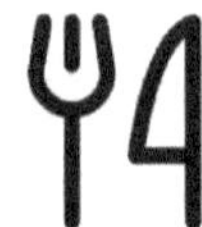
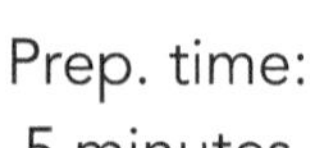

Prep. time:
5 minutes

Cooking time:
15 minutes

Servings:
2

DIRECTIONS:

1. Toasted bagel slices should be golden brown.

2. Spread cream cheese on both sides of the bagel. Season with lemon pepper after adding the onion and tomato slices.

Dilly Scrambled Eggs

INGREDIENTS:

- 2 eggs large
- 1/8 tsp. of black pepper
- 1 tsp. of dried dill
- 1 tbsp. of goat cheese (crumbled)

NUTRITION PER SERVING:

- Calories: 109 Cal
- Protein: 3 g
- Carbs: 7 g
- Fat: 2 g

Prep. time:
5 minutes

Cooking time:
15 minutes

Servings:
4

DIRECTIONS:

1. Before putting the eggs into the pan over medium heat, whisk them in a bowl.
2. Before serving, toss the eggs with black pepper and dill weed.
3. Cook until the eggs are scrambled.
4. Garnish with a dab of goat cheese (crumbled).

Southwest Baked Egg Cups

INGREDIENTS:

- 3 cups of rice, cooked
- 4 oz. of cheddar cheese
- 4 oz. of green chilies
- 2 oz. of pimentos, drained and diced
- 1/2 cup of skim milk
- 2 beaten eggs
- 1/2 tsp. of ground cumin
- 1/2 tsp. of black pepper
- 1 cooking spray (nonstick)

NUTRITION PER SERVING:

- Calories: 109 Cal
- Protein: 5 g
- Carbs: 13 g
- Fat: 4 g

Prep. time:
15 minutes

Cooking time:
35 minutes

Servings:
12

DIRECTIONS:

1. Combine the eggs, cumin, rice, pimentos, milk, cheese, chiles, and pepper in a mixing bowl.

2. Using nonstick cooking spray, coat muffin cups.

3. Fill 12 muffin cups all the way to the top with batter. The remaining 2 oz. of shredded cheese should be sprinkled over each cup.

4. Preheat the oven to approximately 400°F and bake for about 15 minutes, or until done.

Spicy Tofu Scrambler

INGREDIENTS:

- 1 tsp. of olive oil
- 1/4 cup of bell pepper (red)
- 1/4 cup of bell pepper (green)
- 1 cup of firm tofu
- 1 tsp. of onion powder
- 1/4 tsp. of garlic powder
- 1 clove of garlic, minced
- 1/8 tsp. of turmeric

NUTRITION PER SERVING:

- Calories: 213 Cal
- Protein: 18 g
- Carbs: 10 g
- Fat: 13 g

 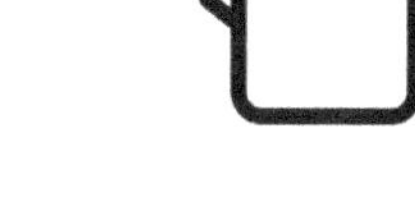 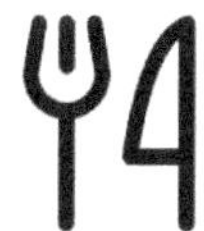

Prep. Time:
5 minutes

Cooking time:
15 minutes

Servings:
2

DIRECTIONS:

1. Sauté garlic and bell peppers in olive oil in a skillet.

2. It is necessary to wash and drain the tofu before breaking it into the pan. In a mixing bowl, combine the other ingredients and whisk well.

3. Cook for approximately 20 minutes, stirring occasionally, or until tofu becomes a light golden color. The water in the mix will evaporate.

4. The tofu scrambler should be heated before serving

Easy Turkey Burritos

INGREDIENTS:

- 1 lb. of ground turkey
- 8, 6-inches of burrito shells (flour)
- 1/4 cup of canola oil
- 8 beaten scrambled eggs
- 1/4 cup of diced onions
- 1/4 cup of bell peppers (fresh)
- 2 tbsps. Of jalapeño peppers (seeded)
- 2 tbsps. Of fresh scallions (chopped)
- 2 tbsps. Of fresh cilantro (chopped)
- 1/2 tsp. of chili powder
- 1/2 tsp. of smoked paprika
- 1 cup of Cheddar cheese (shredded)

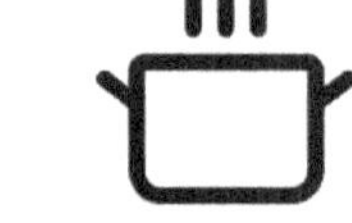

Prep. Time:
10 minutes

Cooking time:
30 minutes

Servings:
4

DIRECTIONS:

1. In half of the oil, sauté the meatloaf, onions, cilantro, scallions, and peppers until transparent. Remove the spices from the fire after tossing them in.

2. Set aside the remaining oil and scrambled eggs in a sauté pan over medium-high heat.

3. Half-fill tortilla shells with vegetable and meatloaf mixture, half-fill with cheddar, half-fill with eggs, fold and serve.

NUTRITION PER SERVING:

- Calories: 407 Cal
- Protein: 25 g
- Carbs: 23 g
- Fat: 3 g

Spiced Salmon a Fusion of Flavors

INGREDIENTS:

- 1/2 cup olive oil for margination
- 2 tbsps. Of olive oil for cooking
- 1/4 cup of lemon juice
- 1 tbsp. of white vinegar
- 1 tbsp. of honey
- 4 tsps. Garlic, minced
- 4 tsps. Ginger, minced
- 1/4 tsp. paprika
- 1/2 tsp. cumin
- 1/2 tsp. chili or pepper powder
- 1/8 tsp. salt
- 2 salmon fillets or 6 oz. each

NUTRITION PER SERVING:

- Calories: 400 Cal
- Protein: 18 g
- Carbs: 12 g
- Fat: 14 g

  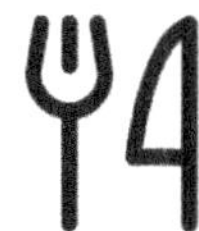

Prep. Time:
35 minutes

Cooking time:
45 minutes

Servings:
4

DIRECTIONS:

1. Whisk the olive oil, honey, lemon juice, spices, and vinegar together in a mixing bowl until the margination is smooth.

2. To make four 3-oz pieces of salmon, cut each salmon fillet in half lengthwise. Pour the margination over the salmon in a mixing bowl, making sure it is well coated.

3. After 30-60 minutes of chilling, remove the bowl from the refrigerator and set it aside to rest at room temperature for 10 minutes before serving.

4. In a skillet pan, heat the oil over medium-high heat until it shimmers. Place the salmon fillets in the pan and fry for 4 minutes on each side, or until the temperature reaches 1450°F.

Easy Summer Pasta Light and Healthy

INGREDIENTS:

- 2 cups rotini noodles, dry
- 1 bell pepper, diced
- 1 onion, diced
- 1 zucchini or summer squash, chopped
- 1 tbsp. of canola oil
- 1/4 cup Parmesan cheese, vegan
- Black pepper according to taste

NUTRITION PER SERVING:

- Calories: 230 Cal
- Protein: 6 g
- Carbs: 8 g
- Fat: 4 g

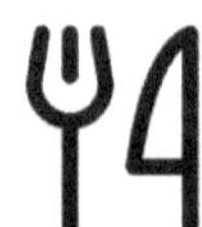

Prep. Time: 10 minutes

Cooking time: 15 minutes

Servings: 4

DIRECTIONS:

1. Bring a big pot halfway full of water to a boil. Cook for around 8-10 minutes, or until the rotini noodles are cooked through.

2. Heat the oil in a skillet over medium heat and cook the pepper, zucchini, and onion until tender.

3. Drain the pasta and toss it in the pan with the veggies.

4. Season with freshly ground black pepper and a sprinkle of vegan Parmesan cheese, if preferred.

Low-Phosphorus Pizza Kid and Kidney-Friendly

INGREDIENTS:

- 1 cup vegan cheese, shredded
- 4 white pitas, small
- 1 bell pepper, red diced
- 8 cherry tomatoes, quartered
- 1 tbsp. of olive oil

NUTRITION PER SERVING:

- Calories: 270 Cal
- Protein: 7 g
- Carbs: 4 g
- Fat: 5 g

Prep. Time:
5 minutes

Cooking time:
10 minutes

Servings:
4

DIRECTIONS:

1. Using a pastry brush, coat the tomatoes and chopped bell pepper in olive oil.

2. Divide the cheese, tomato, and bell pepper among the four pitas equally.

3. Toast for 5 minutes under the broiler in the oven or toaster oven, or until the cheese melts.

Fish Fillets

INGREDIENTS:

- 3 oz. white fish fillets, 2 each
- 1 tbsp. unsalted olive oil or butter, unsalted
- spice blend: 1 tsp. of Mrs Dash
- original and 1 tsp. Mrs Dash
- garlic and herb seasoning

NUTRITION PER SERVING:

- Calories: 103 Cal
- Protein: 3.4 g
- Carbs: 11.7 g
- Fat: 1 g

Prep. Time:
5 minutes

Cooking time:
7 minutes

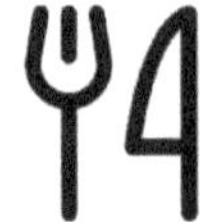

Servings:
2

DIRECTIONS:

1. 1 tbsp. canola oil or unsalted butter, heated in a pan
2. Fish fillets should be put here.
3. Marinate the fish in the spice mixture on both sides.
4. In a heated pan, cook for 3 minutes on each side.
5. Squeeze fresh lemon juice over the fish fillets, according to your liking.

Pasta Salad

INGREDIENTS:

- 2 cups fusilli pasta, cooked
- 1/2 small- diced tomato
- 1/2 red- diced onion
- 1/4 cup olives – pitted and sliced
- 1/2 green bell pepper, sliced
- 1cup cauliflower, chopped

NUTRITION PER SERVING:

- Calories: 69 Cal
- Protein: 2.5 g
- Carbs: 12.5 g
- Fat: 1.3 g

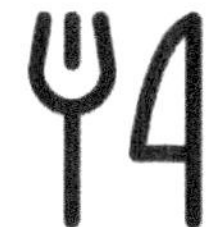

Prep. time: 20 minutes

Cooking time: 50 minutes

Servings: 2

DIRECTIONS:

1. Follow the package instructions for cooking the pasta.
2. In a strainer, rinse the pasta.
3. Vegetables need to be included in the recipe.
4. Toss with a low-fat dressing and serve right away.

Chicken Tortilla Casserole

INGREDIENTS:

- 13 oz. chicken soup condensed cream, reduced-sodium, reduced-fat
- 8 oz. of soy yogurt (plain)
- 1and 1/2 tsp. of chili powder
- 1/3 tsp. cumin
- 1 large, cooked chicken breast
- 8 tortilla, small 4" corn tortillas, (no salt added)
- 1/3 red bell pepper, small
- 1/3 yellow bell pepper, small
- 1/3 orange bell pepper, small
- 3 tbsp. fresh cilantro
- 1 cup sweet yellow corn
- 13 oz canned red tomatoes with green chili
- 1/2 cup reduced-fat Mexican cheese blend
- 1/4 cup of rice milk unsweetened

NUTRITION PER SERVING:

- Calories: 152 Cal
- Protein: 10.6 g
- Carbs: 18.9 g
- Fat: 4.5 g

Prep. time: 35 minutes

Cooking time: 45 minutes

Servings: 8

DIRECTIONS:

1. Preheat the oven to 350°F
   Nonstick cooking spray should be used to coat a 13 by 9-inch baking dish.

2. Peppers that have been chopped should be utilized. Tortillas should be torn into tiny pieces before being used. Chicken that has been shredded should be utilized. Prepare the cilantro by chopping it finely.

3. In a large mixing bowl, mix the soup, the tomatoes, the nondairy yoghurt, the rice milk, the chili powder, the cumin, the chicken, the tortillas, the bell peppers, the corn, and the cilantro.

4. Halfway fill a baking dish with the ingredients.

5. Bake for 40 minutes, covered with Al foil.

6. Remove the lid and sprinkle half a cup of cheese on top of the dish.

7. Cover and bake for 5-10 minutes more, or until the cheese is melted.

8. Allow for 5 minutes of resting time before serving with cilantro.

Chicken Pad Thai

INGREDIENTS:

- 1 lb. rice noodles (look for a low-sodium variety)
- 1/4 cup of vegetable oil
- 1 cup sliced cooked chicken
- 1 Tbsp. garlic, minced
- 4 green onions, sliced on the diagonal
- 1 chili pepper, diced
- 1egg
- 2/3 cup of Pad Thai Sauce
- 1 lime
- 1/8 cup chopped cilantro

NUTRITION PER SERVING:

- Calories: 219 Cal
- Protein: 12 g
- Carbs: 23 g
- Fat: 9 g

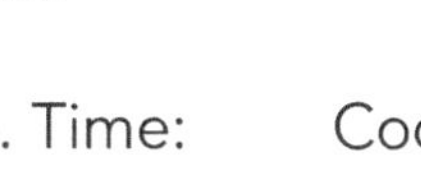

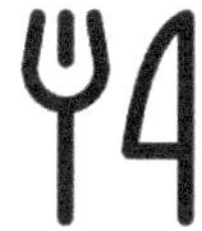

Prep. Time:
30 minutes

Cooking time:
55 minutes

Servings:
3

DIRECTIONS:

1. Soak the rice noodles in water for about 40 minutes

2. Prepare the chicken after that, slice.

3. In a mixing dish, combine all the ingredients for the Pad Thai Sauce.

4. In one-fourth cup vegetable oil, sauté half of the green onion, garlic, and pepper.

5. Toss in some noodles to round off the dish. In a large mixing bowl, combine all the ingredients.

6. Cook the egg until it is fully done.

7. Toss in the Thai sauce to mix. In a large mixing bowl, combine all the ingredients.

8. Add the remaining lime juice and cilantro over the top. Enjoy!

Cowboy Caviar Bean and Rice Salad

INGREDIENTS:

- 1/2 cup cooked, fresh or frozen corn
- 3 cups cooked rice
- 1/4 cup of lime juice
- 1/2 cup canola oil or olive
- 2 tbsps. of brown sugar
- 1 tbsp. of Dijon mustard
- 1/2 tsp. of black pepper
- 1/2 cup diced red bell pepper
- 1/2 cup drained and rinsed, canned black beans, low sodium
- 1 jalapeño, seeded and diced
- 1/2 cup chopped cilantro

NUTRITION PER SERVING:

- Calories: 237 Cal
- Protein: 4 g
- Carbs: 34 g
- Fat: 1 g

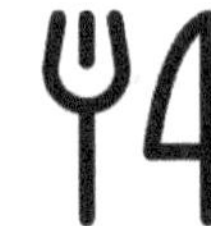

Prep. time: 30 minutes

Cooking time: 50 minutes

Servings: 2

DIRECTIONS:

1. Remove the corn and rice from the heat and place them on a cooling rack.

2. Combine the black pepper, lime juice, mustard, oil, and brown sugar in a mixing bowl to prepare the dressing.

3. Combine the remaining ingredients in a mixing bowl.

4. Toss the salad well in the dressing.

5. Refrigerate for one hour to enable flavors to mingle.

Kickin' Chicken Tacos

INGREDIENTS:

- 1 lb. chicken breasts, skinless and boneless
- 1 1/2 tsps. of salt-free taco seasoning
- 1 lime, juiced
- 8 corn tortillas
- 1 cup chopped or shredded iceberg lettuce
- 1/4 cup of sour cream
- 2 green onions sliced (scallions)
- 1/2 cup chopped cilantro

NUTRITION PER SERVING:

- Calories: 141 Cal
- Protein: 14 g
- Carbs: 9 g
- Fat: 12 g

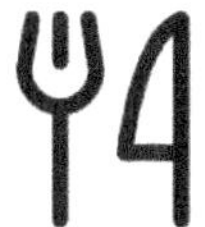

Prep. time:
10 minutes

Cooking time:
30 minutes

Servings:
3

DIRECTIONS:

1. Cook your chicken for around 20 minutes on low heat.
2. Shredded chicken or chunks of chicken should be chewable.
3. Toss the chicken with the Mexican spice and lime juice just before serving.
4. Wrap the lettuce and chicken tightly in the tortillas.
5. Other ingredients like cilantro, sour cream, and green onions may be added if desired.

Herb Breaded Chicken

INGREDIENTS:

- 1/4 tsp. of basil
- 1/4 tsp. of thyme
- 1/4 tsp. of oregano
- 1/4 tsp. of tarragon
- 1/4 tsp. of paprika
- 1/4 tsp. black pepper, fresh ground
- 1 1/2 whole wheat bread, slices
- 1-lb boneless chicken breasts or 1 1/2 lbs. "bone-in" chicken

NUTRITION PER SERVING:

- Calories: 172 Cal
- Protein: 27 g
- Carbs: 7 g
- Fat: 20 g

  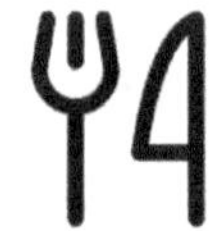

Prep. time:
30 minutes

Cooking time:
1 hour

Servings:
3

DIRECTIONS:

1. Preheat the oven to 400°F.
2. Combine the herbs and spices with the bread in a blender or food processor.
3. Combine all the ingredients well.
4. In a small dish, coat the chicken with the herb mixture.
5. Bake for 20 minutes (for boneless chicken) or 50 minutes (for bone chicken) in a single layer at 350°F (bone-in).

Fruity Chicken Salad

INGREDIENTS:

- 2 cups chicken breasts or 12.5 oz. canned chicken, cooked and cubed
- 1 cup almonds, sliced
- 1 stalk chopped celery,
- 1 chopped green onion
- 2 cups grapes, seedless
- 1 cubed apple
- 3/4 cup raisins
- 1/2 cup of sour cream
- 1/4 cup of mayo
- 1 tsp. unseasoned rice vinegar
- 2 tsps. of sugar
- 1/2 tsp. of Chinese Five-Spice Blend

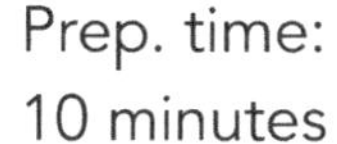  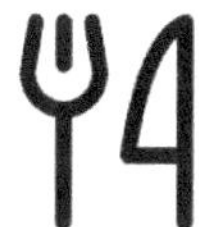

Prep. time:
10 minutes

Cooking time:
30 minutes

Servings:
3

DIRECTIONS:

1. Combine the chicken, raisins, almonds, apples, celery, grapes, and green onion in a large mixing bowl.

2. In a second bowl, whisk together the sour cream, mayonnaise, rice vinegar, Chinese Five-Spice Blend, and sugar until well combined.

3. The chicken mixture and the dressing should be mixed.

NUTRITION PER SERVING:

- Calories: 279 Cal
- Protein: 15 g
- Carbs: 20 g
- Fat: 11 g

Fruity Chicken Salad

INGREDIENTS:

- 4 chicken breasts (boneless)
- 1/4 cup of Dijon mustard
- 3 tbsps. of honey
- 1 tsp. of lemon Juice
- 1 tsp. of curry powder

NUTRITION PER SERVING:

- Calories: 189 Cal
- Protein: 25 g
- Carbs: 14 g
- Fat: 258 mg

Prep. time:
15 minutes

Cooking time:
40 minutes

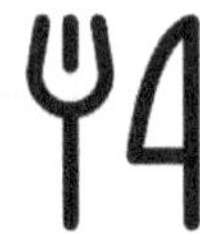

Servings:
4

DIRECTIONS:

1. Preheat the oven to 350°F.

2. In an oven dish, bake the chicken for around 30 minutes

3. In a separate dish, combine the other ingredients.

4. The sauce should be spread on all sides of the chicken.

5. Cook for 30 minutes, or until the internal temperature reaches 165°F, whichever comes first.

Cider Cream Chicken

INGREDIENTS:

- 4 chicken breasts (with bone)
- 2 tbsps. butter, unsalted
- 3/4 cup apple cider
- 1/2 cup half and half

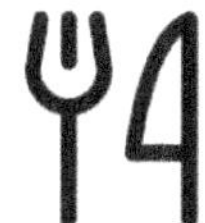
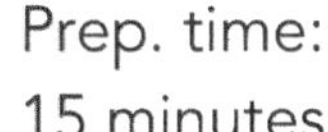

Prep. time:
15 minutes

Cooking time:
40 minutes

Servings:
4

NUTRITION PER SERVING:

- Calories: 186 Cal
- Protein: 27 g
- Carbs: 1 g
- Fat: 20 g

DIRECTIONS:

1. Melt the butter in a medium saucepan over medium-high heat. Place the chicken in the pan and brown on both sides.

2. After adding the apple cider and reducing the heat to medium, cook for about 20 minutes

3. Take the chicken out of the pan and set it aside.

4. Bring the cider to a boil and reduce it to approximately a quarter cup.

5. Stir in half-and-half over low heat until slightly thickened.

6. With a cream sauce, serve the chicken.

Canned Fish Tacos

INGREDIENTS:

- 2 tbsps. onion, chopped
- 2 tsps. oil
- 1 can tuna, drained and rinsed
- 1/2 cup canned or frozen corn
- 1/4 cup canned diced tomatoes (without salt)
- 1/2 tsp. of chili powder
- 4 corn tortillas

NUTRITION PER SERVING:

- Calories: 137 Cal
- Protein: 5 g
- Carbs: 21 g
- Fat: 4 g

Prep. time:
10 minutes

Cooking time:
20 minutes

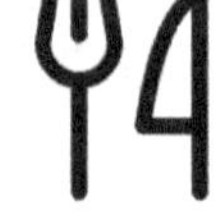

Servings:
4

DIRECTIONS:

1. Over medium heat, sauté the onions in oil until they are transparent.
2. Combine the tuna, chili powder, corn, and tomatoes in a mixing bowl.
3. Cook for another 3-5 minutes, or until the vegetables are at room temperature.
4. Serve with warmed tortillas on the side. If desired, top with lettuce, sour cream, and spicy sauce.

Egg Fried Rice

INGREDIENTS:

- 2 tsps. sesame oil, dark
- 2 eggs
- 2 egg whites
- 1 tbsp. of canola oil
- 1 cup bean sprouts
- 1/3 cup chopped green onions
- 4 cups cold, cooked rice
- 1 cup thawed frozen peas
- 1/4 tsp. black pepper, ground

NUTRITION PER SERVING:

- Calories: 137 Cal
- Protein: 5 g
- Carbs: 21 g
- Fat: 4 g

 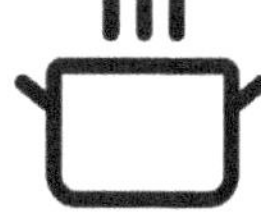

Prep. time:
20 minutes

Cooking time:
35 minutes

Servings:
10

DIRECTIONS:

1. In a mixing bowl, whisk together the egg whites, sesame oil, and eggs; once completely combined, put aside.

2. In a nonstick skillet, heat the canola oil over medium-high heat until it shimmers.

3. Stir in the egg mixture until it is well cooked.

4. Combine the green onion and bean sprouts in a large mixing bowl. Cook for 2 minutes on high heat.

5. Combine the rice and peas in a mixing bowl. Continue to whisk until all the ingredients have reached room temperature.

6. Serve immediately after seasoning with freshly ground black pepper.

Fired-Up Zucchini Turkey Burger

INGREDIENTS:

- 1 lb. turkey meat, ground
- 1 cup shredded zucchini
- 1/2 cup minced onion
- 1 jalapeño pepper, seeded and minced sliced lengthwise
- 1 egg
- 1 tsp. Extra Spicy Blend
- 2 fresh-sliced in half lengthwise and seeded poblano peppers
- 1 tsp. mustard

NUTRITION PER SERVING:

- Calories: 211 Cal
- Protein: 12 g
- Carbs: 25 g
- Fat: 10 g

Prep. time:
10 minutes

Cooking time:
30 minutes

Servings:
4

DIRECTIONS:

1. The first six components must be well combined. With your hands, form four turkey burger patties from the meat mixture. Turkey burgers may be cooked in the oven or grilled on a grill or an electric griddle. Grill the peppers for 5 minutes on each side alongside the turkey patties or until the skin is soft and blistered. The internal temperature should be 165°F when grilling turkey patties or until the center is no longer pink.

2. On a bun, serve the patties with grilled peppers (hamburger).

Turkey Burger

INGREDIENTS:

- 2 tbsps. finely diced jalapeño
- Juice and zest of 2 limes
- 1 tbsp. black pepper, freshly ground
- 1 tbsp. reduced-sodium French's® Worcestershire sauce
- 4 tbsps. olive oil (extra virgin)
- 8 slices mozzarella cheese (plus skim milk)
- 2 lbs. turkey, ground
- 8 toasted hamburger buns

NUTRITION PER SERVING:

- Calories: 211 Cal
- Protein: 12 g
- Carbs: 35 g
- Fat: 10 g

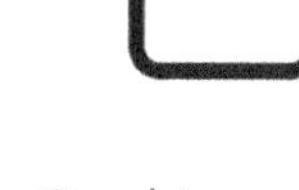

Prep. time:
15 minutes

Cooking time:
35 minutes

Servings:
4

DIRECTIONS:

1. Combine the 1st five ingredients, plus 2 tbsps. olive oil, in a mixing bowl. Brush 2 tbsps. olive oil evenly over equal-sized turkey burger patties.

2. Warm half of the oil in a nonstick sauté pan over medium heat (canola oil).

3. Cook for 6–7 minutes on each side, turning once or until the internal temperature reaches 165° F.

4. Melt approximately 2 tbsp. Cheese on top of the burger in a toaster oven or an oven set to broil.

5. The turkey burger should be served on toasted bread.

Five-Spice Chicken Lettuce Wraps

INGREDIENTS:

- 6 oz. chicken breast, cooked and minced
- 1 scallion, chopped both green and white parts
- 1/2 red apple, chopped and cored
- 1/2 cup bean sprouts
- 1/4 English cucumber, chopped
- 1 lime Juice
- 1 lime Zest
- 2 tbsps. chopped fresh cilantro
- 1/2 tsp. Chinese 5-spice powder
- 8 Boston lettuce leaves

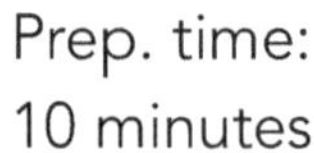  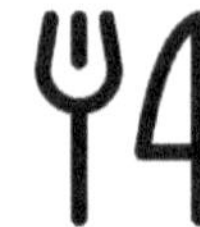

Prep. time:
10 minutes

Cooking time:
30 minutes

Servings:
8

DIRECTIONS:

1. Mix the chicken, cilantro, scallions, lime juice, apple, cucumber, bean sprouts, and five-spice powder in a large mixing bowl.

2. Make an equal distribution of the chicken mixture among the 8 lettuce leaves.

3. Serve the lettuce wrapped around the chicken mixture.

NUTRITION PER SERVING:

- Calories: 407 Cal
- Protein: 32 g
- Carbs: 20 g
- Fat: 22 g

Creamy Pesto Pasta

INGREDIENTS:

- 8-oz, linguine noodles
- 2 cups basil leaves (packed)
- 2 cups arugula leaves (packed)
- 1/3 cup walnut, pieces
- 3 garlic cloves
- 1/4 cup olive oil (extra-virgin)
- Black pepper, to taste (freshly grounded)

NUTRITION PER SERVING:

- Calories: 350 Cal
- Protein: 7 g
- Carbs: 3 g
- Fat: 2 g

Prep. time:
10 minutes

Cooking time:
20 minutes

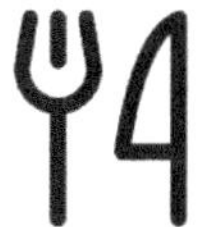

Servings:
4

DIRECTIONS:

1. Bring a half-filled stockpot of water to a boil. Drain the noodles once they've been cooked till they're done.

2. Combine the basil, garlic, arugula, and walnuts in a food processor. Process until the mixture is coarsely ground. While the food processor is running, gently drizzle in the olive oil and blend until smooth. Season with salt and pepper to taste.

3. Before serving, toss the noodles with the pesto.

Crunchy Chicken Salad Wraps

INGREDIENTS:

- 8 oz. chicken, cooked and shredded
- 1 scallion chopped white and green parts
- 1/2 cup halved, seedless red grapes
- 1 celery stalk, chopped
- 1/4 cup Mayonnaise (low sodium)
- A pinch of black pepper, freshly ground
- 4 lettuce leaves (large), red leaf or butter

NUTRITION PER SERVING:

- Calories: 401 Cal
- Protein: 10 g
- Carbs: 45 g
- Fat: 21 g

 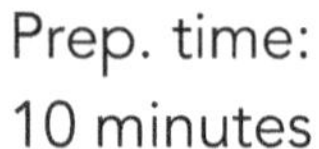  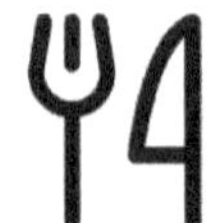

Prep. time:
10 minutes

Cooking time:
10 minutes

Servings:
4

DIRECTIONS:

1. Combine the chicken, mayonnaise, scallion, celery, and grapes in a mixing bowl.

2. Preheat the oven to 350°F. Salt and pepper to taste.

3. To serve, place the chicken salad on top of the lettuce leaves.

Parsley Burger

INGREDIENTS:

- Ground beef, lean, 1 pound
- Black pepper, 1/4 tsp.
- Lemon juice, 1 tbsp.
- Ground thyme, 1/4 tsp.
- Parsley flakes, 1 tbsp.
- Oregano, 1/4 tsp.

NUTRITION PER SERVING:

- Calories: 147 Cal
- Protein: 15 g
- Carbs: 8 g
- Fat: 5 g

  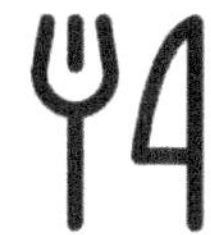

Prep. time:
10 minutes

Cooking time:
15 minutes

Servings:
4

DIRECTIONS:

1. Finely chop all the ingredients.
2. Make 4 tiny equal-sized patties (about 3/4)" thickening
3. Place in a skillet or pan that has been gently oiled.
4. Keep 3 minutes on the broiler "10 to 15 minutes away from the heat, rotating once.

NOTES

5

Dinner Recipes

Crazy Chicken

INGREDIENTS:

- 2 chicken breasts, boneless
- 1/2 diced onion
- 1/2 chopped orange or red bell pepper
- 1/2 yellow or green bell pepper, diced
- 3 garlic cloves
- 1 finely diced carrot
- 1/2 cup broccoli, frozen
- 1/2 green or yellow squash, 1-inch piece each
- 3 tbsp. vegetable or canola oil
- 1/2 tsp. of pepper powder
- 1/4 tsp. of salt

NUTRITION PER SERVING:

- Calories: 180 Cal
- Protein: 19 g
- Carbs: 12.1 g
- Fat: 15 g

Prep. time:
10 minutes

Cooking time:
20 minutes

Servings:
6

DIRECTIONS:

1. Chicken breasts should be cut into 1" pieces.
2. To marinade the chicken breasts, smash the garlic cloves and combine them with the sliced chicken breasts.
3. In a large pan, heat the oil and add the chopped chicken breasts.
4. Cook the chicken until it is golden brown.
5. Cook for 1 minute with the chopped onion before adding the sliced carrots, broccoli, bell peppers, and squash and cook for another 6 minutes
6. Salmon may be substituted for the chicken in this meal if desired.

Turkey Paprika

INGREDIENTS:

- 1 chopped onion
- 1/2 cup of mushrooms
- 3 tbsp. unsalted butter
- 2 tbsp. of flour
- 2 tsp. of paprika powder
- 1 cup reduced-sodium chicken broth or turkey
- 2 lightly beaten egg yolks
- 1 cup of sour cream
- 2 cups of sliced cooked turkey
- 1/2 cup cooked rice or noodles per person
- 2 tbsp. unsalted butter
- 1 tsp. of poppy seeds

NUTRITION PER SERVING:

- Calories: 519 Cal
- Protein: 34.5 g
- Carbs: 24 g
- Fat: 0 g

Prep. time:
10 minutes

Cooking time:
30 minutes

Servings:
4-5

DIRECTIONS:

1. Melt butter in a pot and cook mushrooms and onions until soft.
2. After adding the salt, paprika, and flour, pour in the liquid.
3. Cook for 1 minute, constantly stirring, until the liquid thickens and bubbles form.
4. Once a little quantity of the hot mixture has been mixed into the egg yolks, return to the heated mixture.
5. Cook for another minute on low heat.
6. Whisk in the sour cream until it is completely smooth.
7. On top of it, place the turkey.
8. Reduce the heat to a low setting until it reaches a comfortable temperature.
9. As a side dish, serve with rice or noodles.
10. Toss with 2 tbsp. unsalted butter and 1 tsp. poppy seeds just before serving.

Thai Pizza

INGREDIENTS:

- 1 recipe of readymade Pizza Dough
- 1/2 - 1 cup of diced chicken, cooked
- 1/2 cup of peanut sauce
- 3 stalks of chopped green onion
- 8-10 leaves of fresh basil
- 1 cup grated mozzarella cheese

NUTRITION PER SERVING:

- Calories: 309 Cal
- Protein: 19 g
- Carbs: 31 g
- Fat: 0 g

 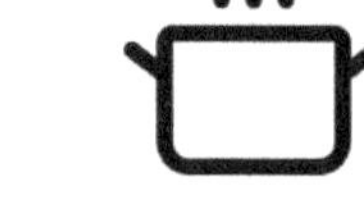

Prep. time: 5 minutes

Cooking time: 15 minutes

Servings: 8

DIRECTIONS:

1. Preheat the oven to 500°F.

2. Roll out the pizza dough to a thickness of 1/4 inch and a diameter of 12-14 inches.

3. Assemble the peanut sauce and distribute it to the visitors.

4. Combine basil, chicken, and green onion in a mixing bowl.

5. Serve with a cheese sprinkle on top.

6. Preheat oven to 350°F and bake for 8 to 12 minutes

Szechuan Shrimp

INGREDIENTS:

- 6 tbsp. of oil
- 1/4 tsp. crushed ginger root
- 3 chopped garlic cloves
- 1 lb. peeled shrimps
- 1 tbsp. of sugar
- 3 tbsp. of sherry wine
- 1 tsp. of hot sauce
- 1 tsp. low sodium Soy Sauce
- 2 tbsp. ketchup without salt
- 1/2 cup minced scallions
- 1 tbsp. of cornstarch
- 3 tbsp. of water

NUTRITION PER SERVING:

- Calories: 318 Cal
- Protein: 16 g
- Carbs: 11 g
- Fat: 0 g

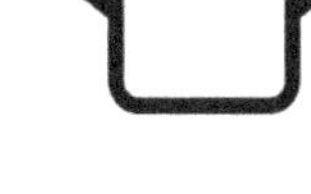

Prep. time:
10 minutes

Cooking time:
15 minutes

Servings:
4

DIRECTIONS:

1. In a pan, heat the oil and sauté the garlic and ginger root until light brown.

2. Combine the sherry, sugar, shrimp, scallions, low sodium soy sauce, ketchup, and hot pepper sauce in a mixing bowl.

3. 10 minutes of frying and combining

4. To thicken the shrimp mixture, whisk together cornstarch and water.

Quick Fettuccine

INGREDIENTS:

- 1/2 – 2/3 cup of boiling water
- 1 pack of penne pasta
- 2-3 chopped cloves garlic
- 1 tsp. of canola oil
- 1 cup of fish, shrimp, or meat of choice
- 1-2 cups of veggies (peas, broccoli, asparagus)
- 1 package of cream cheese or Neufchatel
- 1/2 cup shredded parmesan cheese
- 1/4 cup of fresh parsley
- 1/4 cup basil, fresh

NUTRITION PER SERVING:

- Calories: 304 Cal
- Protein: 18 g
- Carbs: 32 g
- Fat: 0 g

  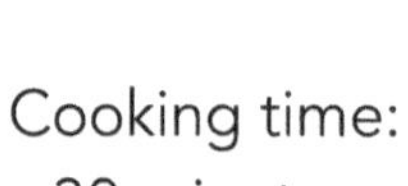

Prep. time: 15 minutes

Cooking time: 30 minutes

Servings: 6

DIRECTIONS:

1. Bring the water for the pasta to a boil.
2. Remove approximately 2 cups of boiling water once the water has come to a simmer and add the pasta.
3. In a frying pan, sauté garlic in oil while waiting for the water to boil.
4. If you're adding meat or vegetables, sauté them in a pan with garlic until they're done.
5. Combine fresh herbs, cheeses, and half a cup of hot water in a food processor or blender.
6. Add more water if the sauce is too thick.
7. Pour over vegetables/meat and sautéed garlic in a frying pan, if desired.
8. Pour the sauce over the noodles.

Oven-Fried Chicken

INGREDIENTS:

- 1/4 cup unsalted butter
- 1/4 cup of corn oil
- 1/2 cup of flour
- 1/2 cup of cornmeal
- 1 tbsp. of paprika powder
- 1 tsp. powdered ground pepper
- 1 tsp. crushed mustard
- 1 tbsp. tarragon, dried
- 1 tbsp. marjoram, dried
- 4 lb. whole chicken, sliced

NUTRITION PER SERVING:

- Calories: 376 Cal
- Protein: 24 g
- Carbs: 15 g
- Fat: 0 g

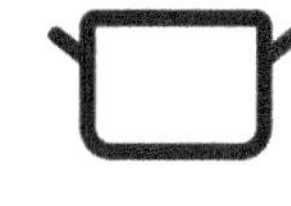

Prep. time:
15 minutes

Cooking time:
25 minutes

Servings:
8

DIRECTIONS:

1. Preheat the oven to 425°F.
2. In the bottom of a 9x13 inch pan, melt 1/4 cup unsalted butter and 1/4 cup oil.
3. Melt the butter and oil in an oven-safe pan.
4. Fill a plastic bag with 12 cups cornmeal and 1/2 cup flour while the oil and butter mixture are melting.
5. To taste, season with salt and pepper.
6. Give it a thorough shake after adding the chicken pieces.
7. Place the chicken pieces in the heated oil, skin side down.
8. Preheat the oven for around thirty minutes
9. Cook for another 20 to 30 minutes on the other side.

Mediterranean Pizza

INGREDIENTS:

- 2 readymade pita bread or pizza dough
- 1 tbsp. extra virgin olive oil
- 2 chopped garlic cloves
- 1 diced tomato, sliced
- 10 thinly chopped basil leaves
- 3 oz. ricotta or goat cheese

NUTRITION PER SERVING:

- Calories: 176 Cal
- Protein: 7 g
- Carbs: 18 g
- Fat: 0 g

Prep. time:
10 minutes

Cooking time:
30 minutes

Servings:
12

DIRECTIONS:

1. Preheat the oven to 450°F.

2. The pizza crust should be brushed with olive oil.

3. Garlic should be spread evenly over the crust.

4. Tomato slices should be used to cover the garlic cloves.

5. After the basil, evenly sprinkle the goat cheese over the pie.

6. Bake for 10-15 minutes in the oven, or according to the crust package Instructions.

Orange-Glazed Chicken

INGREDIENTS:

- 1/4 cup canola oil
- 6 boneless chicken breasts cut into halves
- 2 tbsp. of flour
- 1/8 tsp. of nutmeg
- 1 chunk ginger
- 1/4 tsp. of cinnamon
- 1 1/2 cup fresh orange Juice
- 1/4 cup of raisins
- 1/2 cup of mandarin orange

NUTRITION PER SERVING:

- Calories: 262 Cal
- Protein: 24 g
- Carbs: 15 g
- Fat: 3 g

Prep. time:
30 minutes

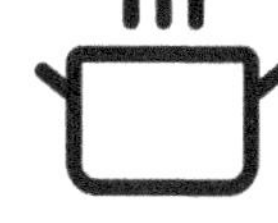

Cooking time:
55 minutes

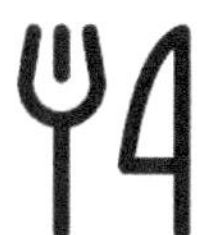

Servings:
6

DIRECTIONS:

1. In a nonstick pan, heat some oil.
2. All sides of the chicken should be done.
3. removing the chicken from the pan
4. Combine the ginger, flour, nutmeg, and cinnamon in a mixing bowl; add the heated oil.
5. To prepare a smooth paste, whisk everything together rapidly.
6. Slowly pour the orange juice into the pan.
7. Constantly stir.
8. Cook for 3 minutes over medium heat, stirring periodically, or until soft and thickened.
9. Toss the chicken back into the pan.
10. Cook over low heat for approximately 30 minutes or until the chicken is soft and cooked through.
11. If the sauce is too thick, thin it down with water.
12. Heat till hot, then add the mandarin orange slice.

Italian Meatballs

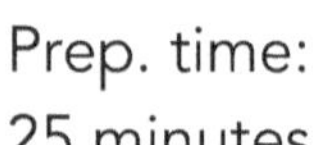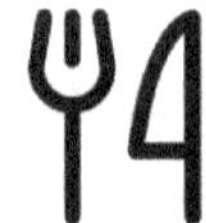

Prep. time:
25 minutes

Cooking time:
45 minutes

Servings:
2

INGREDIENTS:

- 1 lb. ground beef
- 2 large, whisked eggs
- 1/2 cup of oatmeal, dried
- 3 tbsp. grated parmesan cheese
- 1/2 tbsp. extra virgin olive oil
- 1/2 tbsp. of garlic powder
- 1 tsp. oregano, dried
- 1/2 cup diced onion
- 1/2 tsp. of powdered black pepper

NUTRITION PER SERVING:

- Calories: 120 Cal
- Protein: 12 g
- Carbs: 13 g
- Fat: 10 g

DIRECTIONS:

1. Preheat the oven to 375°F.

2. In a mixing bowl, whisk together all the ingredients well.

3. Form the dough into 1-inch balls and place it on a baking pan.

4. Cook for a further 10-15 minutes, or until the meatballs are cooked through.

5. Before serving, reheat the meatballs in a dish or a skillet over low heat. 2 tbsp. Sauce (served separately) Make use of red pepper. To enhance taste, make a roasted sauce.

Fruit Vinegar Chicken

INGREDIENTS:

- 2 lb. Chicken
- 1/2 cup of berry or fruit vinegar
- 1/4 cup of canola oil
- 1/4 cup fresh orange juice
- 1/2 tsp. of marjoram
- 1/2 tsp. crushed basil
- 1/2 tsp. of tarragon

NUTRITION PER SERVING:

- Calories: 163 Cal
- Protein: 13 g
- Carbs: 4 g
- Fat: 2 g

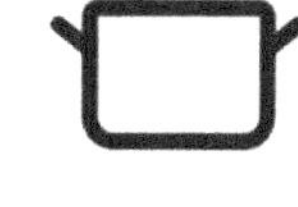

Prep. time:
15 minutes

Cooking time:
20 minutes

Servings:
6

DIRECTIONS:

1. Preheat the oven to 350°F.
2. In a big zip lock bag, combine all the ingredients.
3. Allow the marinade to cool for 15 to 20 minutes
4. Place the chicken on the baking sheet after removing it from the bag.
5. Bake for 30 minutes, or until the chicken reaches an internal temperature of 165°F.

Fast Roast Chicken with Lemon & Herbs

INGREDIENTS:

- 1 whole chicken, defrosted
- 2 tbsp. of softened butter
- 2 1/2 tbsp. diced fresh herbs (parsley, thyme)
- 2 minced garlic cloves
- 1 small, diced lemon
- 1 tbsp. of extra virgin olive oil

NUTRITION PER SERVING:

- Calories: 413 Cal
- Protein: 28 g
- Carbs: 3 g
- Fat: 2 g

Prep. time:
30 minutes

Cooking time:
40 minutes

Servings:
4-6

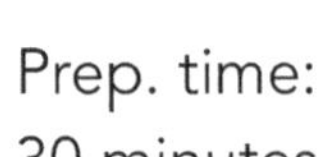

DIRECTIONS:

1. Preheat the oven to 450°F.
2. In a roasting pan, place the chicken.
3. In a small mixing bowl, combine the herbs, butter, and garlic.
4. Place the herbed butter and lime wedges in the cavity of the chicken.
5. Apply olive oil to the bird's skin.
6. Roast for 15 minutes per pound of meat, or until an internal temperature of 165°F is reached.
7. Pour the buttery liquids and lemon wedges over the chicken.
8. Allow the chicken to rest for 20 minutes before cutting.

Dilled Fish

INGREDIENTS:

- 1 1/2 lb. white fish, fresh
- 1 tsp. crushed onions (dried)
- 1/4 tsp. of mustard powder
- 1/2 tsp. of dill weed
- Pepper to taste
- 4 tsp. of fresh lemon juice

NUTRITION PER SERVING:

- Calories: 251 Cal
- Protein: 19 g
- Carbs: 0 g
- Fat: 0 g

Prep. time:
15 minutes

Cooking time:
50 minutes

Servings:
6

DIRECTIONS:

1. Preheat the oven to 475°F.
2. After washing the fish, rinse it and pat it dry.
3. Combine all the ingredients in a baking dish.
4. Combine the pepper, dill weed, two tbsps. of water, onion, and mustard in a mixing dish.
5. Toss the spice with the lemon juice and pour evenly over the fish.
6. Bake for 17-20 minutes, covered.

Pasta with Cheesy Meat Sauce

INGREDIENTS:

- 1/2 box pasta
- 1 lb. minced beef
- 1/2 cup chopped onions
- 1 tbsp. of onion flakes
- 11/2 cups low sodium beef stock
- 1 tbsp. Bouillon® beef with no salt
- 1 tbsp. unsalted tomato sauce
- 3/4 cup grated pepper jack or Monterey cheese
- 8 oz. cream cheese, soft
- 1/2 tsp. of Italian seasoning
- 1/2 tsp. black pepper powder
- 2 tbsp. of Worcestershire sauce

NUTRITION PER SERVING:

- Calories: 112 Cal
- Protein: 23 g
- Carbs: 1 g
- Fat: 3 g

Prep. time:
25 minutes

Cooking time:
30 minutes

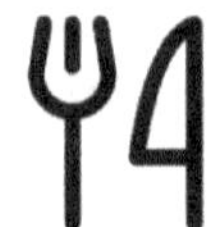

Servings:
6

DIRECTIONS:

1. Cook the pasta according to the package instructions.

2. Cook the ground beef with the onions and onion flakes in a large pan.

3. Combine the tomato sauce, stock, and bouillon in a mixing bowl.

4. Reduce the heat to low and continue to cook, stirring periodically. Turn off the heat and add the cooked pasta, grated cheese, softened cream cheese, and spices (Italian seasoning, Worcestershire sauce, and black pepper) in a large mixing bowl. Stir the cheese into the pasta mixture until it is completely melted.

Crunchy Green Bean Casserole

INGREDIENTS:

- 12 oz. green beans, fresh
- 2 tbsp. of hot sauce
- 1/4 cup grated cheddar cheese or gorgonzola
- 2 tbsp. unsalted butter, melted
- 1/2 cup breadcrumbs
- 2 tbsp. of diced green onions
- 1/2 cup of crumbled tortilla chips, plain

NUTRITION PER SERVING:

- Calories: 502 Cal
- Protein: 23 g
- Carbs: 35 g
- Fat: 30 g

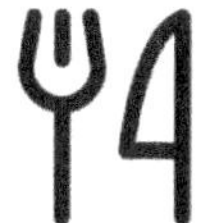

Prep. time:
15 minutes

Cooking time:
25 minutes

Servings:
6

DIRECTIONS:

1. Preheat the oven to 375°F.

2. Green beans should be chopped into 2-inch pieces and mixed with the spicy sauce in a mixing dish (boil for 5–7 minutes on a microwave-safe pan with a wet moist paper towel). Fill a casserole dish halfway with the ingredients.

3. In a small mixing dish, combine the remaining ingredients. Sprinkle evenly over string green beans before serving, and bake uncovered for 12–15 minutes, or until desired crispness is reached.

Slow-Cooked Lemon Chicken

INGREDIENTS:

- 1 tsp. of dried oregano
- 1/4 tsp. crushed black pepper
- 2 tbsp. of unsalted butter
- 1 lb. skinless and boneless chicken breast
- 1/4 cup of reduced-sodium chicken broth
- 1/4 cup of water
- 1 tbsp. fresh lemon juice
- 2 chopped garlic cloves
- 1 tsp. diced fresh basil

NUTRITION PER SERVING:

- Calories: 122 Cal
- Protein: 4 g
- Carbs: 11 g
- Fat: 6 g

Prep. time: 2 hours

Cooking time: 5 hours

Servings: 4

DIRECTIONS:

4. In a mixing dish, combine oregano and black pepper. The chicken should be coated with the mixture.

5. In a saucepan over medium heat, melt the butter. Transfer the chicken to the slow cooker after frying it in the melted butter.

6. In a saucepan, combine the water, garlic, chicken broth, and lemon juice. Bring it to a moderate simmer to loosen the browned pieces stuck to the bottom of the pan. Pour the sauce over the chicken.

7. Cook for 2.5 hours with the lid on. Cook for 5 hours over medium-high heat or 5 hours in a slow cooker.

8. Sprinkle the basil over the chicken and baste it. Cook for a further 15–30 minutes on high, or until chicken is well cooked.

Chili Cornbread Casserole

INGREDIENTS:

Chili:

- 1 lb. ground beef
- 1/2 cup of chopped onions
- 1/4 cup chopped celery
- 2 tbsp. diced jalapeño
- 1/2 cup diced green/red peppers
- 1 tbsp. of chili powder
- 1 tbsp. garlic powder
- 2 tbsp. onion flakes, dried
- 1 tbsp. cumin powder
- 1 tsp. freshly ground pepper
- 1/2 cup of tomato sauce without salt
- 1/4 cup of water
- 1/4 cup Worcestershire sauce (low sodium)
- 1 cup washed and drained kidney beans
- 1 cup grated cheddar cheese

Cornbread:

- 1/4 cup of cornmeal
- 3/4 cup of whole-wheat flour
- 1/4 tsp. of baking soda
- 1/2 tsp. of cream
- 1/2 cup brown sugar
- 1 beaten egg
- 11/2 tbsp. unsalted butter, melted
- 1/4 cup of canola/olive oil
- 3/4 cup of milk

 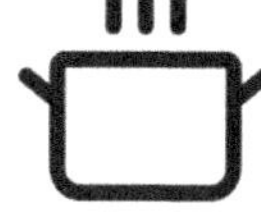 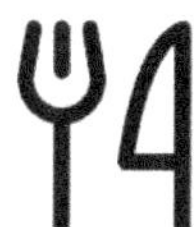

Prep. time:
25 minutes

Cooking time:
30 minutes

Servings:
8

DIRECTIONS:

1. Combine the minced brown meat, onions, jalapenos, celery, and bell peppers in a large saucepot. It's a good idea to drain any oil that isn't being utilized. Chili powder, onion flakes, beans, garlic powder, cumin, water, tomato sauce, black pepper, and Worcestershire sauce should all be added at this point. Cook for another 10 minutes.
Remove the cheese from the skillet and place it on a 9" 9" baking sheet.
2. Combine the sugar, cornmeal, baking soda, flour, and cream of tartar in a medium mixing bowl.
3. In a small bowl, whisk together the milk, oil, egg, and melted butter. Combine the flour and egg mixture (some lumps are fine; do not overbeat).
4. Pour the mixture over the chili and bake for 25 minutes uncovered, then 20 minutes covered before turning off the oven and letting it rest for 5 minutes

NUTRITION PER SERVING:

- Calories: 197 Cal
- Protein: 26 g
- Carbs: 1 g
- Fat: 9 g

Spaghetti and Asparagus Carbonara

INGREDIENTS:

- 2 tsp. of canola oil
- 1 cup chopped onions
- 1 large beaten egg
- 1 cup of cream
- 1/4 cup of chicken stock with low sodium
- 3 cups of noodle pasta, cooked
- 2 cups diced asparagus, fresh
- 1 tsp. of freshly ground black pepper
- 1/2 cup diced scallions.
- 3 tbsp. of meatless bacon bits
- 3 tbsp. grated Parmesan cheese

NUTRITION PER SERVING:

- Calories: 392 Cal
- Protein: 17 g
- Carbs: 33 g
- Fat: 21 g

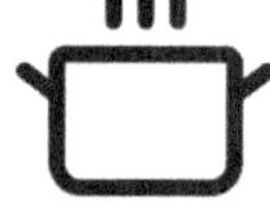

Prep. time:
25 minutes

Cooking time:
55 minutes

Servings:
6

DIRECTIONS:

1. Heat the oil over medium heat in a large nonstick pan and sauté the chopped onions until lightly browned.

2. Whisk the egg and cream together in a mixing dish until well combined.

3. Reduce the heat to low and pour the cream slowly into the onions, stirring continuously with a wooden spatula until the cream thickens approximately 4–6 minutes

4. Stir for 3–4 minutes more, or until the black pepper, stock, pasta, and asparagus are well heated.

5. Remove the carbonara from the heat and place it on a platter to serve. Serve with onions, bacon, and cheese on top.

Chicken and Gnocchi Dumplings

INGREDIENTS:

- 2 lb. boneless chicken breast
- 1 lb. of gnocchi
- 1/4 cup of olive oil or grapeseed oil
- 1 tbsp. of chicken base (reduced sodium)
- 6 cups chicken broth (low sodium)
- 1/2 cup of thinly diced celery
- 1/2 cup thinly chopped onions
- 1/2 cup diced carrots, fresh
- 1/4 cup diced parsley
- 1 tsp. of black pepper powder
- 1 tsp. of Italian seasoning

NUTRITION PER SERVING:

- Calories: 304 Cal
- Protein: 9 g
- Carbs: 27 g
- Fat: 19 g

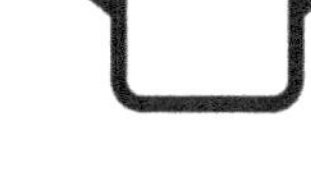

Prep. time: 15 minutes

Cooking time: 50 minutes

Servings: 10

DIRECTIONS:

1. Put the stockpot on the stove, add the oil, and bring it to a high temperature.

2. Cook the chicken in a skillet until golden brown on both sides.

3. With the chicken, cook until the celery, carrots, and onions are transparent. Cook for 20 to 30 minutes over high heat with chicken stock.

4. Reduce heat to low and whisk in black pepper, chicken bouillon, and Italian seasoning after adding the gnocchi. Cook and stir continuously for 15 minutes

5. After removing the pan from the heat and garnishing with chopped parsley, serve immediately.

Smoking Good Chicken with Mustard Sauce

INGREDIENTS:

- 2 lb. skinless and boneless chicken breasts finely diced
- 1/4 cup of shallots slices
- 1/4 cup diced scallions, fresh
- 1/2 cup of flour
- 1/2 cup oil
- 2 cups chicken stock (reduced sodium)
- 2 tbsp. brown mustard
- 1/2 stick of chilled butter, cubed

Seasonings:

- 1/2 tsp. of black pepper powder
- 1/2 tsp. of Italian Seasoning
- 1 tbsp. of parsley, dried
- 1 tbsp. of smoked paprika

NUTRITION PER SERVING:

- Calories: 362 Cal
- Protein: 28 g
- Carbs: 38 g
- Fat: 10 g

Prep. time: 20 minutes

Cooking time: 1 hours

Servings: 8

DIRECTIONS:

1. In a mixing bowl, combine paprika, pepper, Italian seasoning, and parsley.
2. The chicken fillet is dusted with half of the flour, and the remainder is stirred in.
3. Fill a broad saucepan halfway with water and set it aside. Heat the oi in it.
4. Set aside three tbsps. of seasoned flour.
5. Cook the chicken for 2-3 minutes on each side after covering it in the remaining seasoned flour.
6. Remove the chicken from the pan and place it on a cooling rack. Remove everything except a few tbsps. of oil from the pan, add the shallots, and cook until they are slightly transparent.
7. Whisk in the flour until smooth, then trickle in the stock in a slow, steady stream while whisking. Reduce heat to low and whisk in unsalted butter, mustard, and chicken bouillon after 5 minutes of simmering over medium-high heat.
8. Turn off the heat and return the chicken and any liquid drippings from the dish to the pan, stirring constantly. Serve with scallions on top.

Pesto-Crusted Catfish

INGREDIENTS:

- 2 lbs. catfish fillets
- 4 tsp. of pesto
- 3/4 cup breadcrumbs
- 1/2 cup shredded mozzarella cheese
- 2 tbsp. extra virgin olive oil
- Chef McCargo's Signature Seasoning Blend:
- 1 tsp. of garlic powder
- 1 tsp. powdered onion
- 1/2 tsp. of dried oregano leaves
- 1/2 tsp. of red chili flakes
- 1/2 tsp. of black pepper powder

NUTRITION PER SERVING:

- Calories: 361 Cal
- Protein: 28 g
- Carbs: 9 g
- Fat: 23 g

Prep. time:
20 minutes

Cooking time:
40 minutes

Servings:
6

DIRECTIONS:

1. Preheat the oven to 400°F.

2. In a small mixing bowl, combine all the spices and sprinkle evenly over both sides of the salmon.

3. Set aside equal quantities of pesto on the top side of the fillets.

4. Combine the breadcrumbs, cheese, and oil in a medium mixing bowl, then dredge the pesto side of the fish in the mixture until fully covered.

5. Place the fish pesto on a baking sheet pan that has been well oiled or coated with oil, allowing space between the fillets.

6. Bake on the bottom rack for 15 to 20 minutes at 400°F, or until desired brownness is achieved.

7. Allow 10 minutes for the fish to rest after removing it from the dish to avoid it breaking.

Hawaiian-Style Slow-Cooked Pulled Pork

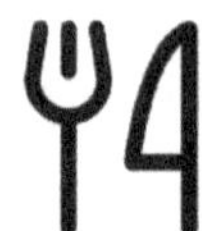

Prep. time:
50 minutes

Cooking time:
5 hours

Servings:
16

INGREDIENTS:

- Pork roast, 4 pounds
- Black pepper, 1/2 tsp., freshly ground
- Paprika, 1/2 tsp.
- Onion powder, 1 tsp.
- Garlic powder, 1/2 tsp.
- Liquid smoke, 2 tbsp.
- Pickled or radishes red onions (optional garnish)

NUTRITION PER SERVING:

- Calories: 312 Cal
- Protein: 26 g
- Carbs: 15 g
- Fat: 16 g

DIRECTIONS:

1. Combine paprika, black pepper, garlic powder, and onion in a small container.

2. Season the pork on both sides with the spice mix. Place the meat in a slow cooker or crock-pot. Add some liquid smoke to the mix.

3. Fill the crock-pot or slow cooker with enough water to reach a depth of 14–12 inches. Cook on high for 4–5 hours

4. Remove the pork from the cooker and shred it with two forks.

Pasta with Cheesy Meat Sauce

INGREDIENTS:

- Pasta, large-shaped, 1/2 box
- Ground beef, 1 pound
- Onions, 1/2 cup, diced
- Onion flakes, 1 tbsp.
- Beef stock, 1 1/2 cups, reduced-sodium
- Beef bouillon, 1 tbsp., no salt added
- Tomato sauce, 1 tbsp., no salt added
- Pepper jack or Monterey cheese, 3/4 cup shredded
- Cream cheese, 8 oz, softened
- Italian seasoning, 1/2 tsp.
- Black pepper, 1/2 tsp., ground
- Worcestershire sauce, 2 tbsp., reduced sodium

NUTRITION PER SERVING:

- Calories: 285 Cal
- Protein: 20 g
- Carbs: 1 g
- Fat: 21 g

Prep. time: 45 minutes

Cooking time: 55 minutes

Servings: 6

DIRECTIONS:

1. Cook the pasta according to the package instructions.

2. In a large skillet, brown the ground meat. Fry until the meat is well-browned, adding onion flakes and onions as needed.

3. Drain the noodles and combine the browned meat with the bouillon, stock, and tomato sauce.

4. Cook, often stirring, until the mixture begins to boil. Remove from heat and stir in shredded cheese, softened cream cheese, and spices (black pepper, Italian seasoning, and Worcestershire sauce).

5. Mix the spaghetti with the meat mixture until the cheese is completely melted.

Spicy Beef Stir-Fry

INGREDIENTS:

- Cornstarch, 2 Tbsp., separated
- Sesame oil, 1/4 tsp.
- Sugar, 1/2 tsp.
- Water, 2 Tbsp., separated
- Egg, 1 large, beaten
- Canola oil, 3 Tbsp., separated
- Beef round tip, 12 oz, sliced
- Bell pepper, 1 green, sliced
- Onions, 1 cup, sliced
- Red chili pepper, 1/4 tsp., ground (or to taste)
- Sherry, 1 tbsp.
- Soy sauce, 2 tsp., reduced-sodium
- Parsley (optional garnish)

NUTRITION PER SERVING:

- Calories: 502 Cal
- Protein: 23 g
- Carbs: 35 g
- Fat: 30 g

Prep. time:
25 minutes

Cooking time:
45 minutes

Servings:
4

DIRECTIONS:

1. Combine 1 tbsp. cornstarch, 1 large egg, 1 tbsp. canola oil, 1 tbsp. water, and the meat in a large mixing bowl. Allow for a 20-minutes rest period.

2. Combine the remaining water and cornstarch in a separate dish.

3. Heat the remaining 2 tbsps. of oil in a pan and add the marinated beef mixture. Cook until the meat is golden brown.

4. Combine the onion, green bell peppers, and chili pepper in a large mixing bowl. Drizzle the sherry over everything and stir-fry for a minute. Combine the sesame oil, sugar, and soy sauce in a mixing bowl.

5. Mix the cornstarch and water and pour it in. Serve after stirring until it thickens.

Homemade Pan Sausage

INGREDIENTS:

- Cooking spray
- Ground pork,1pound, fresh lean (or beef)
- Granulated sugar, 2 tsp.
- Ground black pepper, 1 tsp.
- Ground sage, 2 tsp.
- Ground red pepper, 1/2 tsp.
- Basil, 1 tsp. (optional)

NUTRITION PER SERVING:

- Calories: 261 Cal
- Protein: 21 g
- Carbs: 10 g
- Fat: 15 g

 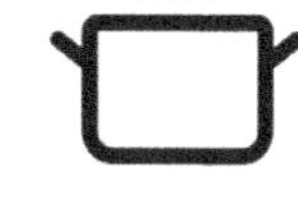 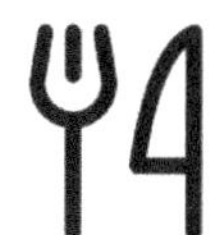

Prep. time:
30 minutes

Cooking time:
25 minutes

Servings:
12

DIRECTIONS:

1. To prepare sausage, thoroughly combine all ingredients.

2. To prepare a patty, take 2 tbsp. of the meat mixture and shape it into a patty.

3. Broil or pan fry until fully done.

Open-Faced Steak & Onion Sandwich

INGREDIENTS:

- Chopped steaks, 4, (4-ozs each)
- Lemon juice, 1 tbsp.
- Italian seasoning, 1 tbsp.
- Black pepper, 1 tbsp.
- Vegetable oil, 1 tbsp.
- Onion, 1 medium, sliced into rings
- Herbed bread,4 slices

NUTRITION PER SERVING:

- Calories: 22 Cal
- Protein: 6 g
- Carbs: 1 g
- Fat: 7 g

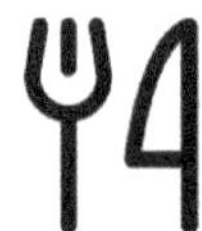

Prep. time:
30 minutes

Cooking time:
40 minutes

Servings:
2

DIRECTIONS:

1. Black pepper, Italian spice, and lemon juice are used to season the meat.

2. Heat the oil in a sauté pan over medium heat.

3. Season steaks with salt and pepper and cook until browned on both sides and tender. Drain on paper towels after removing from pan.

4. Reduce heat to low, add the onion, and cook until soft.

5. Serve open-faced on herbed bread with onion rings on top.

Chili Rice with Beef

INGREDIENTS:

- Vegetable oil, 2 tbsp.
- Ground beef, 1 pound, lean
- Onion, 1 cup, chopped
- Rice, 2 cups, cooked
- Chili con carne seasoning powder, 1 1/2 tsp.
- Black pepper, 1/8 tsp.
- Sage, 1/2 tsp.

NUTRITION PER SERVING:

- Calories: 360 Cal
- Protein: 23 g
- Carbs: 26 g
- Fat: 14 g

 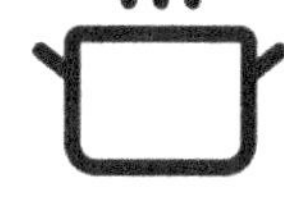

Prep. time: 25 minutes

Cooking time: 50 minutes

Servings: 4

DIRECTIONS:

1. Heat the oil in a pan and add the meat and onion. Fry, stirring regularly, until golden brown.

2. Season the cooked rice with salt and pepper. Combine the two.

3. Remove yourself from the heat. Cover with a lid and let aside for 10-14 minutes before serving.

Jalapeno Pepper Chicken

INGREDIENTS:

- Vegetable oil, 3 tbsp.
- Chicken, cut up, 2-3 pounds (skin and fat removed)
- Onion,1, sliced into rings
- Chicken bouillon, low sodium, 1 1/2 cups
- Ground nutmeg, 1/2 tsp.
- Black pepper, 1/4 tsp.
- Jalapeño peppers, 2 tsp., fresh, chopped finely, and seeded

NUTRITION PER SERVING:

- Calories: 143 Cal
- Protein: 17 g
- Carbs: 2 g
- Fat: 7 g

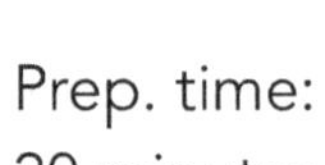

Prep. time:
20 minutes

Cooking time:
55 minutes

Servings:
8

DIRECTIONS:

1. Cook the chicken pieces in a large pan with oil over medium-high heat until golden. Set aside and keep heated.

2. In a heated skillet, put brown onion rings. Add the bouillon and bring to a boil, constantly stirring.

3. Return the chicken to the pan and season with black pepper and nutmeg. Cover and cook for 35 minutes, or until chicken is tender.

4. Cook on low for the next minute after adding the jalapeno peppers.

Crispy Oven Fried Chicken

INGREDIENTS:

- Fryer chicken, 2 1/2 pounds, (cut as desired)
- Lemon juice, 1 tbsp.
- All-purpose flour, 1 cup
- Black pepper, 1 tsp.
- Corn flakes, 1 cup, crushed
- Poultry seasoning, 1/4 tsp.
- Vegetable oil, 4 tbsp.

NUTRITION PER SERVING:

- Calories: 280 Cal
- Protein: 15 g
- Carbs: 15 g
- Fat: 18 g

Prep. time: 30 minutes

Cooking time: 60 minutes

Servings: 8

DIRECTIONS:

1. Preheat the oven to 400°F.

2. Rinse the chicken pieces well and dry them with a kitchen towel before massaging them with lemon juice.

3. In a small bag, combine flour, corn flakes, poultry spice, and black pepper. Give it a good shake.

4. Use vegetable oil to oil a shallow baking pan (about "deep").

5. Place the chicken in the bag containing the flour and spice mixture, big chunks first. Give it a good shake.

6. In an oiled pan, place the coated chicken.

7. Bake for 20-30 minutes on each side, or until golden brown.

Barbecue Cups

INGREDIENTS:

- Ground turkey, 3/4 pounds lean
- Spicy barbecue sauce, 1/2 cup
- Onion flakes, 2 tsp.
- Garlic powder, dash
- Refrigerator biscuits, low-fat, 1 10-oz package

NUTRITION PER SERVING:

- Calories: 134 Cal
- Protein: 7 g
- Carbs: 13 g
- Fat: 5 g

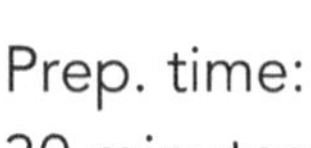

Prep. time: 30 minutes

Cooking time: 40 minutes

Servings: 10

DIRECTIONS:

1. Cook the turkey in a nonstick pan until it is golden brown.

2. Combine the garlic powder, barbecue sauce, and onion flakes in a mixing bowl. Mix everything up well.

3. Oil muffin pans, flatten one biscuit, and place one at a time into muffin tins.

4. Spoon the meat mixture into the middle of each biscuit cup.

5. Preheat the oven to 400°F and bake for around 10 to 12 minutes

Turkey & Noodles

INGREDIENTS:

- Elbow macaroni, 2 cups dry
- Vegetable, 1 tbsp. (or olive oil)
- Lean ground turkey, 2 pounds fresh
- Green onions, 1/2 cup, chopped
- Green pepper, 1/2 cup, chopped
- Regular tomatoes, 1 14-oz can, diced
- Italian seasoning, 1 tbsp.
- Black pepper, 1 tsp.

NUTRITION PER SERVING:

- Calories: 273 Cal
- Protein: 33 g
- Carbs: 22 g
- Fat: 7 g

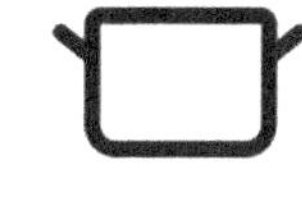

Prep. time:
20 minutes

Cooking time:
35 minutes

Servings:
6

DIRECTIONS:

1. Begin by bringing a big pot of water to a boil, then adding the macaroni. Allow to boil for 5 minutes or until desired tenderness is reached. Drain and set aside the macaroni.

2. Heat the vegetables in a large skillet. Heat the oil over a medium flame. Add the ground turkey to the hot oil and cook until done, stirring regularly.

3. Cooked macaroni, chopped tomatoes, green peppers, onions, black pepper, and Italian seasoning all mixed well.

4. Cook for another 5 minutes, covered. Warm the dish before serving.

Easy Turkey Sloppy Joes

INGREDIENTS:

- Red onion, 1/2 cup
- Ground turkey, 7% fat, 1-1/2 pounds
- Bell pepper green, 1/2 cup
- Chicken grilling seasoning blend, 1 tbsp.
- Brown sugar, 2 tbsp.
- Worcestershire sauce, 1 tbsp.
- Tomato sauce, 1 cup, low-sodium
- Hamburger buns, 6

NUTRITION PER SERVING:

- Calories: 290 Cal
- Protein: 24 g
- Carbs: 28 g
- Fat: 9 g

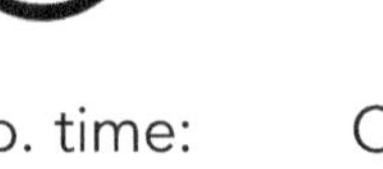

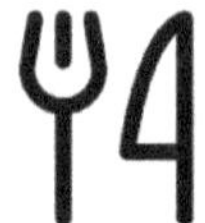

Prep. time:
15 minutes

Cooking time:
55 minutes

Servings:
6

DIRECTIONS:

1. Chop the onion and bell pepper.

2. In a big cast-iron skillet, Cook the veggies with the ground turkey over medium-high heat until the turkey is fully done. The liquid should not be drained.

3. Combine the brown sugar, grilling spice, tomato sauce, and Worcestershire sauce in a small bowl.

4. Toss the beef mixture with the sauce mentioned above. Reduce the heat to low and cook for 10 minutes

5. Serve the turkey mixture on burger buns in six portions.

Chicken and Summer Vegetable Kebabs

INGREDIENTS:

- Olive oil, 2 tbsp.
- Peach jam, 1 tbsp.
- Lemon juice, 2 tbsp.
- Herb seasoning blend, 1 tsp.
- Salt, 1/4 tsp.
- Chicken thighs, boneless, skinless, 1 pound
- Zucchini, 1 medium
- Summer squash, 1 medium, yellow
- Bell pepper, 1 red
- Onion, 1 medium

NUTRITION PER SERVING:

- Calories: 284 Cal
- Protein: 24 g
- Carbs: 10 g
- Fat: 16 g

Prep. time: 20 minutes

Cooking time: 25 minutes

Servings: 6

DIRECTIONS:

1. To prepare the marinade, measure the peach jam into a small microwave-safe dish and liquefy for 10 to 15 seconds in the microwave. Combine the herb seasoning, olive oil, lemon juice, and salt in a mixing bowl. Mix well until everything is fully combined.

2. Wash the chicken thighs and wipe them dry with a paper towel. Each boneless thigh should be cut into four pieces and placed in a zip-lock bag.

3. Toss the boneless pieces with half of the marinade. (The other half of the marinade will be used on the vegetables.) Close the zip-lock bag and marinate it in the refrigerator.

4. To prepare kebabs, slice the vegetables into tiny pieces. Place them in a jar with the rest of the marinade. Toss the vegetables in the mixture to coat them.

5. Using skewers, thread the chicken and veggies together (8 small or 4 large skewers).

6. Place the skewers on a heated medium grill and cook for 12 to 15 minutes with the lid closed. Turn the skewers regularly to ensure even cooking.

Chicken Nuggets with Honey Mustard Dipping

INGREDIENTS:

- Yellow mustard, 1 tbsp.
- Mayonnaise, 1/2 cup
- Honey, 1/3 cup
- Worcestershire sauce, 2 tsp.
- Chicken breasts, 1 pound, boneless
- Low-fat milk, 1%, 2 tbsp.
- Cornflakes, 3 cups
- Egg, 1 large

NUTRITION PER SERVING:

- Calories: 164 Cal
- Protein: 9 g
- Carbs: 14 g
- Fat: 8 g

Prep. time:
20 minutes

Cooking time:
45 minutes

Servings:
12

DIRECTIONS:

1. Combine the mayo, mustard, Worcestershire sauce, and honey in a mixing bowl. Refrigerate the sauce until the nuggets are done, then use it as a dipping sauce.

2. Preheat the oven to 400°F.

3. Cut the breasts into 36 pieces of the same size.

4. Squash the cornflakes and place them in a large zip-lock bag.

5. In a small mixing dish, whisk the egg, then add the milk. Dip the tiny chicken pieces in the whisked egg, then place in a Ziplock bag with the cornflake crumbs and shake to coat.

6. Place the nuggets on a baking sheet coated with nonstick cooking spray and bake for around 15 minutes or soft.

Easy Chicken and Pasta Dinner Sauce

INGREDIENTS:

- chicken, 2-1/2 oz
- vegetables, 2/3 cup
- 1/2 cup red bell pepper
- 1 cup zucchini
- 1 tbsp. olive oil
- 2 cups cooked pasta, any shape
- 5 oz cooked chicken breast
- 3 tbsp. low-sodium Italian dressing

NUTRITION PER SERVING:

- Calories: 400 Cal
- Protein: 30 g
- Carbs: 45 g
- Fat: 11 g

Prep. time:
25 minutes

Cooking time:
30 minutes

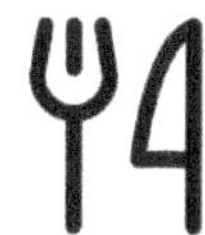

Servings:
2

DIRECTIONS:

1. Bell pepper and zucchini should be sliced.

2. Heat the olive oil in a nonstick skillet and sauté the peppers and zucchini until crispy tender. Remove to a platter.

3. Meat should be cut into strips.

4. Microwave chicken strips and cooked spaghetti one at a time.

5. Toss the spaghetti with the dressing. Serve with chicken strips and veggies that have been sautéed.

6. Adjust the amount of chicken in this meal if you need a higher or lower protein diet.

Stuffed Green Peppers

INGREDIENTS:

- Vegetable oil, 2 tbsp.
- Turkey, 1/2 pound ground and lean (or chicken)
- Onions, 1/4 cup, chopped
- Celery, 1/4 cup, chopped
- Lemon juice, 2 tbsp.
- Celery seed, 1 tbsp.
- Italian seasoning, 2 tbsp.
- Black pepper, 1 tsp.
- Sugar, 1/2 tsp.
- Cooked rice, 1 1/2 cups
- Paprika
- Green peppers, 6 smalls, seeded with tops removed

NUTRITION PER SERVING:

- Calories: 131 Cal
- Protein: 9 g
- Carbs: 15 g
- Fat: 4 g

Prep. time:
20 minutes

Cooking time:
45 minutes

Servings:
6

DIRECTIONS:

1. Preheat your oven to around 325°F.

2. Heat the oil in a saucepan.

3. Cook until the onions, ground beef, and celery are soft and brown.

4. In a saucepan, combine all ingredients except the paprika and green peppers. Remove from the heat and mix everything.

5. Fill peppers halfway with the cooked mixture. Cover it with foil or place it in a baking dish.

6. Preheat your oven to 350°F and bake for around 30 minutes Remove from the pan and season with some paprika.

NOTES

6

Desserts Recipes

Easy Cream Cheese Pumpkin Pie

INGREDIENTS:

- 15 oz. pumpkin pie filling
- 8 oz. light cream cheese
- 8 oz. light cool whip
- 1 tsp. pumpkin pie spice
- 2 crackers, graham
- 1 tsp. cinnamon
- 2 tbsp.

NUTRITION PER SERVING:

- Calories: 227 Cal
- Protein: 3 g
- Carbs: 9 g
- Fat: 1 g

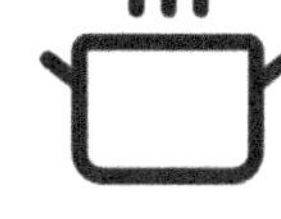

Prep. time:
5 minutes

Cooking time:
10 minutes

Servings:
16

DIRECTIONS:

1. In a stand mixer, beat together the cream cheese, pumpkin, and pie spice until smooth.

2. Gently fold in 8 oz. cool whip to keep the mixture foamy.

3. Half-fill the pie shells with the filling.

4. Check to see whether the crust has been filled.

5. Cover and chill for 1 hour.

6. To serve, drizzle 2 tbsps. cool, whip over each piece and sprinkle with cinnamon.

Old Fashioned Oatmeal Cookies

INGREDIENTS:

- 1 box cake mix spice
- 2 cup oats
- 2 eggs
- 3/4 cup vegetable oil
- 1/2 cup milk
- 1/4 cup chopped nuts
- 1/4 cup dark brown sugar

NUTRITION PER SERVING:

- Calories: 113 Cal
- Protein: 2 g
- Carbs: 30 g
- Fat: 1 g

 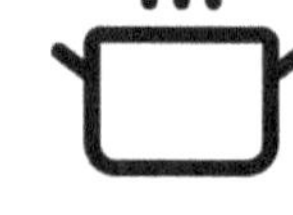

Prep. time:
10 minutes

Cooking time:
22 minutes

Servings:
48

DIRECTIONS:

1. Combine oats, cake mix, eggs, milk, oil, almonds, and sugar in a mixing bowl.

2. 1 tbsp. of the mixture must be put on a regular baking sheet.

3. Preheat the oven to 350°F and bake for 10 to 12 minutes, or until a toothpick inserted in the center comes out clean.

4. Allow the cookies to cool on a cooling rack or a baking sheet.

Peach Cobbler

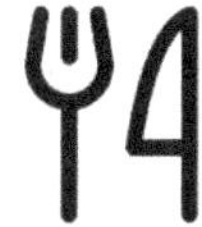

Prep. time:	Cooking time:	Servings:
15 minutes	40 minutes	6

INGREDIENTS:

- 1/2 cup plain flour
- 1/2 cup sugar
- 1/2 cup milk or coffee creamer
- 1 tsp. baking powder
- 2 cup sliced peaches with juice

NUTRITION PER SERVING:

- Calories: 143 Cal
- Protein: 2 g
- Carbs: 25 g
- Fat: 1 g

DIRECTIONS:

1. Combine the sugar, plain flour, and baking powder in a mixing bowl.
2. Mix in the milk or coffee creamer well.
3. In a mixing dish, combine the peaches and their juice.
4. Allow cooling on a baking sheet.
5. Cook for 35 minutes at 350°F, or until the top is thick and golden brown.

Raw Apple Cake

INGREDIENTS:

- 1/2 cup sugar
- 1 cup shortening
- 2 beaten eggs
- 2 cup flour
- 2 tsp. baking soda
- 2 tsp. cinnamon
- 1 tsp. cloves
- 3/4 cup raisins
- 2 cup diced apples
- 1 cup sour cream
- 1 cup diced nuts
- 1 cup cold coffee

NUTRITION PER SERVING:

- Calories: 416 Cal
- Protein: 6 g
- Carbs: 52 g
- Fat: 8 g

  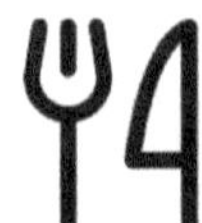

Prep. time: 35 minutes

Cooking time: 50 minutes

Servings: 12

DIRECTIONS:

1. Brush a baking pan with butter and flour before using.

2. Before baking, preheat the oven to 350°F.

3. Combine sugar, flour, shortening, beaten eggs, baking soda, cloves, cinnamon, raisins, sour cream, diced apples, cold coffee, and nuts in a large mixing bowl.

4. Preheat the oven to 350°F and bake the mixture for 60 minutes

5. Before serving, let for complete cooling.

Grandma's Blueberry Cupcakes

INGREDIENTS:

- 1/3 cup shortening
- 1/2 tsp. salt
- 1 tsp. vanilla
- 1 cup sugar
- 1 egg
- 2 1/2 tsp. baking powder
- 2 cups sifted flour
- 3/4 cup milk
- 1 cup blueberries
- Frosting (optional)
- 3 cups grounded sugar
- 1/2 cup butter, unsalted
- 1 tsp. vanilla extract
- 1 tbsp. vanilla

NUTRITION PER SERVING:

- Calories: 162 Cal
- Protein: 3 g
- Carbs: 12 g
- Fat: 1 g

Prep. time:
10 minutes

Cooking time:
30 minutes

Servings:
18

DIRECTIONS:

1. Preheat the oven to 400°F before beginning to bake. Using cupcake liners, line a 12-count muffin tray, then another pan with six liners.

2. Combine the egg, shortening, salt, vanilla, and sugar in a hand mixer. Combine the flour and baking powder in a separate container. After that, gently add the flour and milk mixture to the shortening mixture.

3. Hand-swirl the berries into the batter.

4. After filling muffin pans with batter, bake for around 15-18 minutes

5. Frosting (optional): Using a hand mixer, beat together the butter and icing sugar. Combine the almond milk and vanilla essence in a blender and blend until smooth. Frost the cooled blueberry cupcakes with this.

Lemon Almond Cheesecake A Holiday Favorite

  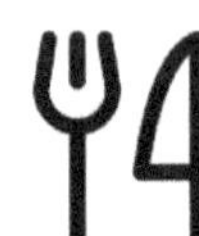

INGREDIENTS:

- 1 1/2 cups crushed graham crackers
- 1 1/2 cups sugar
- 1 1/2 tbsp. sugar
- 6 tbsps. unsalted melted butter
- 2 1/2 lb. cream cheese
- 5 large eggs
- 1 cup sour cream
- 1 tsp. almond extract
- 1 tsp. lemon zest
- 1/2 tsp. vanilla extract

NUTRITION PER SERVING:

- Calories: 440 Cal
- Protein: 7 g
- Carbs: 78 g
- Fat: 3 g

Prep. time:
2 hours

Cooking time:
3 hours

Servings:
15

DIRECTIONS:

1. Preheat the oven to 350°F before baking.
2. Combine the crushed graham crackers (1 1/2 cups), sugar (1 tbsp.), and unsalted melted butter (6 tbsps.) in a mixing bowl, then press into a round cake pan.
3. It should be baked for 10 minutes and then set aside to cool.
4. Combine the cream cheese (2 1/2 pound), sugar (1/2 cup), sour cream (1/4 cup), five eggs, almond extract (1 tsp.), and lemon zest (1 tsp.) in a large mixing bowl and whisk until frothy. Pour the ingredients into the previously prepared crust.
5. Bake for no more than 1 hour, then cool for 4 hours.
6. Serve with a dollop of sour cream on top of the cheesecake.

Rainbow Crispy Treats Fun and Colorful

INGREDIENTS:

- 6 tbsp. unsalted butter
- 10 oz. small marshmallows
- 1 tsp. vanilla extract
- 6 cups rice cereal, crispy
- 1/4 cup rainbow-colored sprinkles

NUTRITION PER SERVING:

- Calories: 200 Cal
- Protein: 1 g
- Carbs: 65 g
- Fat: 0 g

  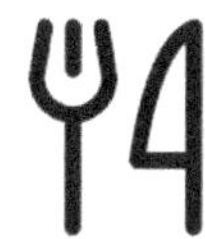

Prep. time:
25 minutes

Cooking time:
35 minutes

Servings:
12

DIRECTIONS:

1. Set aside a baking pan that has been oiled.

2. Melt the butter in a large saucepan over low heat.

3. 1 tsp. vanilla essence and 1 bag of tiny marshmallows, mixed in until marshmallows are completely melted

4. Stir in the crunchy rice cereal and rainbow confetti after removing the pan from the heat. I levelled the mixture in a baking pan.

5. Allow 1 hour for chilling before slicing into 12 even pieces.

Cinnamon Sugar Cookies

INGREDIENTS:

- 2 3/4 cups flour
- 1 1/2 cups sugar
- 1 cup unsalted butter
- 1 tsp. baking soda
- 2 tsp. tartar cream
- 1/2 tsp. almond extract
- 1/2 tsp. vanilla extract
- 2 tsp. cinnamon
- 2 tbsp. brown sugar

NUTRITION PER SERVING:

- Calories: 181 Cal
- Protein: 2 g
- Carbs: 6 g
- Fat: 0 g

Prep. time:
5 minutes

Cooking time:
8-10 minutes

Servings:
24

DIRECTIONS:

1. Preheat the oven to 400°F before baking.

2. Combine the cinnamon and brown sugar in a bowl and put it aside.

3. In a blender, combine all the ingredients (excluding the cinnamon and brown sugar mix).

4. Form the dough into 24 1-inch balls.

5. Coat the balls with a cinnamon and brown sugar mixture.

6. Bake for 8-10 minutes on a baking sheet.

Cinnamon Scented Applesauce

INGREDIENTS:

- 1 lb. apples, Granny Smith
- 1 lb. Fuji apples
- 2 tbsp. lemon juice
- 1/4 cup sugar
- 1/2 tsp. cinnamon
- 1/4 tsp. nutmeg
- 3/4 cup water

NUTRITION PER SERVING:

- Calories: 129 Cal
- Protein: < 1 g
- Carbs: 34 g
- Fat: < 1 g

Prep. time: 10 minutes

Cooking time: 30 minutes

Servings: 5

DIRECTIONS:

1. Apples that have been peeled and cored should be chopped.

2. Combine all the ingredients in a pot and bring to a boil over high heat.

3. Reduce the heat to low and continue to simmer for another 20-30 minutes, or until the liquid has evaporated and the apples have started to cling to the pan's edges.

4. Remove the skillet from the heat and mash the apples to desired consistency with a fork or a potato masher in a food processor.

5. It may be served either warm or cold.

Coconut Holiday Balls

INGREDIENTS:

- 2 cups sugar, Confectioners
- 5 tbsp. cocoa powder
- 1 tsp. ground Allspice
- 1 cup coconut milk
- 2 tbsp. corn syrup
- 1/3 cup brandy or rum
- 5 cups vanilla wafers
- 1 cup shredded coconut

NUTRITION PER SERVING:

- Calories: 270 Cal
- Protein: 2 g
- Carbs: 41 g
- Fat: 11 g

Prep. time:
10 minutes

Cooking time:
15 minutes

Servings:
30

DIRECTIONS:

1. Combine 2 cups confectioners' sugar, cocoa powder, and allspice in a mixing dish.

2. Combine the corn syrup, coconut milk, and rum or brandy in a mixing bowl.

3. Crush the wafers in a food processor until coarsely crushed. Toss them in the sweet mixture and give them a good stir.

4. With your hands, combine the ingredients until they are crumbly and wet. Spread the crushed coconut in a shallow dish.

5. Make 30 one-inch balls with them. Coat each ball with crushed coconut.

Rice Pudding

INGREDIENTS:

- 2 tbsp. butter, unsalted
- 6 tbsps. Carolina rice or jasmine rice
- 1/2 tsp. grounded saffron
- 1/2 tsp. crushed cardamom
- 6 cups milk
- 6 tbsp. brown sugar
- 1/2 cup slivered almonds
- 1/4 cup thinly sliced raw pistachios

NUTRITION PER SERVING:

- Calories: 218 Cal
- Protein: 7 g
- Carbs: 23 g
- Fat: 12 g

 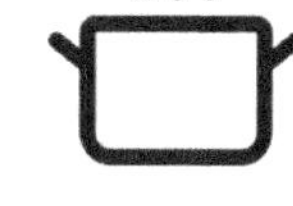

Prep. time:
40 minutes

Cooking time:
1 hour

Servings:
10

DIRECTIONS:

1. In a 10-inch skillet, melt butter over medium heat.

2. After adding the cardamom, rice, and saffron, cook for 2 minutes.

3. Cook for 90 minutes, or until the milk has reduced by half and the rice is mushy, stirring occasionally.

4. Cook for approximately 2 minutes, or until the sugar melts, stirring constantly; add the sugar, almonds, and half of the pistachios.

5. Serve in a serving dish with the remaining pistachios on top.

Vegan Banana Bread

INGREDIENTS:

- 4 medium-sized ripe bananas
- 1/3 cup vegetable oil
- 1/2 cup sugar
- 1/8 tsp. salt
- 1/2 cup applesauce
- 1 1/2 tsp. vanilla extract
- 4 tbsp. crushed flax seeds
- 1 tsp. baking soda
- 2 tbsp. agave nectar
- 1 1/2 cups wheat flour

NUTRITION PER SERVING:

- Calories: 200 Cal
- Protein: 3 g
- Carbs: 33 g
- Fat: 7 g

Prep. time:
30 minutes

Cooking time:
45 minutes

Servings:
12

DIRECTIONS:

1. Before you start baking, preheat your oven to 350°F.

2. Mash the peeled bananas with a fork, then stir in the vegetable oil with a wooden spoon.

3. In a separate mixing dish, combine all the ingredients.

4. Mix in the flour well. Combine all the ingredients in a large mixing bowl and stir until well combined. Half-fill an oiled loaf pan with batter.

5. Cook for 60 minutes, or until the surface gently depresses when pressed. Allow cooling on a cooling rack.

Vegan Chocolate Mousse

INGREDIENTS:

- 1 medium avocado
- 2 tbsp. cacao powder
- 2 tsps. vanilla extract
- 1/4 cup agave syrup
- 1/4 cup oat milk
- 1/4 cup raspberries
- 12 sliced raspberries for garnish
- 1 tbsp. crushed sugar

NUTRITION PER SERVING:

- Calories: 200 Cal
- Protein: 2 g
- Carbs: 37 g
- Fat: 6 g

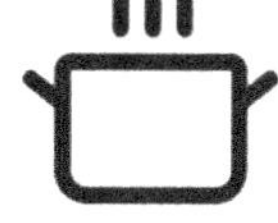

Prep. time:
25 minutes

Cooking time:
45 minutes

Servings:
4

DIRECTIONS:

1. Remove the stone from the avocados by cutting them lengthwise.

2. Using a spoon, scoop out the contents of each half and place them in the food processor.

3. Combine the remaining ingredients in a blender. Blend the ingredients until it is completely smooth.

4. Before serving, chill for at least one hr.

5. Garnish with cut raspberries and powdered sugar.

Stewed Cinnamon Apples

INGREDIENTS:

- 1 tbsp. butter, vegan
- 4 medium-sized peeled apples (cut into eight wedges)
- 1 tsp. crushed cinnamon
- 1/4 cup water
- 1 tbsp. frozen or Greek vanilla yogurt (optional)

NUTRITION PER SERVING:

- Calories: 117 Cal
- Protein: 0.5 g
- Carbs: 25 g
- Fat: 3 g

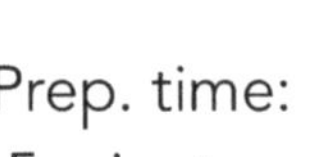

Prep. time:
5 minutes

Cooking time:
12 minutes

Servings:
4

DIRECTIONS:

1. Melt the butter in a large pan over medium heat.

2. In a mixing dish, combine the chopped apples and cinnamon.

3. Reduce the heat to a low setting and pour in the water. Cook, occasionally stirring, for 5-7 minutes, or until the apples are soft.

4. Allow the apples to cool completely before serving with Greek or frozen yogurt.

Watermelon Ice Cream

INGREDIENTS:

- 2/3 cup coconut milk
- 2 medium frozen bananas
- 1/4 tsp. vanilla extract
- Pinch sea salt
- 1 tbsp. honey
- 3 cups cubed watermelon
- Ice cream toppings (optional)

NUTRITION PER SERVING:

- Calories: 99 Cal
- Protein: 1 g
- Carbs: 24 g
- Fat: 1 g

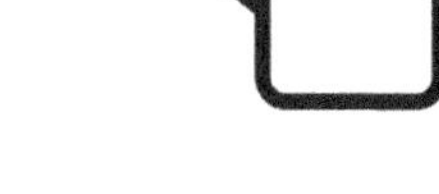

Prep. time:
5 minutes

Cooking time:
15 minutes

Servings:
4

DIRECTIONS:

1. In a bowl, combine the ingredients and pour into the empty ice cube molds or a baking dish.

2. Refrigerate the ingredients for 3 hours or until it has solidified.

3. Fill the blender halfway with frozen watermelon and blend until the mixture is smooth and creamy.

4. Freeze the mixture for approximately 25 minutes in a tight container or until it achieves a thick consistency.

5. Serve it with your favorite toppings, just like ice cream.

Coco Grapes

INGREDIENTS:

- 1/2 lb. concord or other small grapes
- 4 oz. gluten-free semisweet chocolate
- 2 tbsp. cocoa powder, unsweetened

NUTRITION PER SERVING:

- Calories: 145 Cal
- Protein: 2 g
- Carbs: 24 g
- Fat: 7 g

 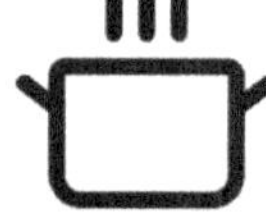

Prep. time: 10 minutes

Cooking time: 15 minutes

Servings: 5

DIRECTIONS:

1. Combine the washed and drained grapes in a mixing dish.
2. Melt the chocolate in a double boiler over medium heat or in the microwave for 30 seconds at a time until it is softened, stirring after each interval.
3. Preheat the oven to 350°F and prepare a baking sheet with parchment paper.
4. 1 tbsp. Melted chocolate drizzled over the grapes, well mixed with a wooden spoon Clean the dish's borders, then swirl the mixture through the middle to evenly coat all the grapes.
5. Allow the chocolate to set before using a fine sieve to sprinkle it with cocoa powder.
6. As you sift, lightly toss the grapes. Pour the chocolate over the grapes and toss to coat and separate them evenly.
7. Using a spatula, spread the mixture onto the baking sheet. Before serving as a dessert or snack, chill for 1-2 hours or until chocolate has set.

Tropical Frozen Yogurt Bars

INGREDIENTS:

- 1/4 cup heavy cream
- 14 oz. Greek yogurt, non-fat
- 1 tbsp. honey
- 1/3 cup coconut chips
- 1/4 cup chocolate chips
- 1/3 cup pineapple pieces
- 1/3 cup mango pieces
- 1 sliced kiwi

NUTRITION PER SERVING:

- Calories: 134 Cal
- Protein: 6 g
- Carbs: 14 g
- Fat: 7 g

Prep. time:
5 minutes

Cooking time:
15 minutes

Servings:
8

DIRECTIONS:

1. Beat the cream into the thick and creamy frosting using a hand mixer.

2. In a second medium mixing dish, combine the yoghurt and the other ingredients (except the kiwi).

3. In a mixing dish, combine the whipped cream and yoghurt mixture.

4. Fill the dish halfway with the mixture, then top with kiwi slices in an attractive design.

5. Refrigerate until the dish is solid.

6. Remove the frozen food from the freezer 10 minutes before serving.

7. Cut the cake into 8 'bars' with a wet knife and serve right away.

Fuyu Persimmon Fruit Salad

INGREDIENTS:

- 2 cups fresh peeled and chopped Fuyu persimmon
- 2 cups fresh and chopped mango
- 5 pitted and chopped Medjool dates
- 4 tbsp. fresh lime juice
- 5 tbsp. pomegranate seeds

NUTRITION PER SERVING:

- Calories: 76 Cal
- Protein: 18 g
- Carbs: 27 g
- Fat: 16 g

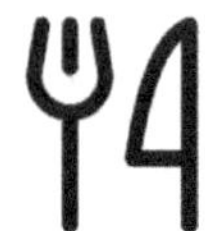

Prep. time:
10 minutes

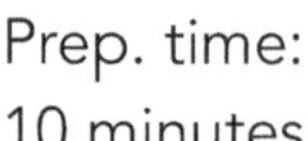

Cooking time:
15 minutes

Servings:
5

DIRECTIONS:

1. In a mixing bowl, combine the persimmon, mango, and dates.

2. Lemon juice should be squeezed and well combined.

3. Add 1 tbsp. pomegranate molasses to each bowl.

Cocadas

INGREDIENTS:

- 2 large egg whites
- 1/3 cup coconut sugar
- 3 cups unsweetened shredded coconut
- 1/4 tsp. baking powder
- 1/2 tbsp. vanilla extract
- 1/2 cup condensed milk, sweetened
- 2 tbsp. chocolate chips
- 1 tsp. coconut oil

NUTRITION PER SERVING:

- Calories: 76 Cal
- Protein: 18 g
- Carbs: 27 g
- Fat: 16 g

Prep. time:
10 minutes

Cooking time:
25 minutes

Servings:
12

DIRECTIONS:

1. Preheat the oven to 350°F before baking.

2. In a medium mixing bowl, whisk egg whites until frothy.

3. Everything, including the shredded coconut, sugar coconut, and baking powder, should be blended. After that, sprinkle in the vanilla extract and condensed milk slowly.

4. Drop approximately 2 tsp. of batter onto a parchment-lined baking sheet at a time to make 12 cocadas.

5. Preheat the oven to 350°F and bake for 15-20 minutes, or until golden brown.

6. Microwave the chocolate chips and coconut oil for 20 seconds on high, then whisk until smooth.

7. Using a spoon, drizzle it over the cooked cocadas.

8. Cocadas may be served at room temperature or heated.

Quick Mini Strawberry Cream Cheese Brownie

INGREDIENTS:

- 1 chocolate fudge brownie
- 2 tsp. whipped strawberry cream cheese
- 1 fresh and sliced strawberry
- 1/2 piece unsweetened white chocolate

NUTRITION PER SERVING:

- Calories: 131 Cal
- Protein: 3 g
- Carbs: 24 g
- Fat: 8 g

 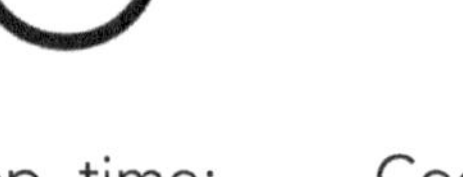 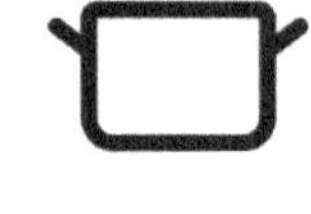 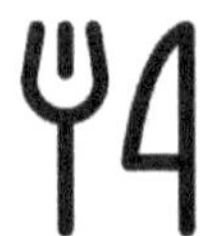

Prep. time:
5 minutes

Cooking time:
5 minutes

Servings:
1

DIRECTIONS:

1. Cut the brownie in half and place 1 tsp. cream cheese on the bottom, another slice on top, and 1 tsp. cream cheese on the bottom.

2. Strawberry slices should be arranged on top.

3. Microwave on high for 30 seconds, stirring after each 30-seconds interval. Microwave for another 5-10 seconds if required.

4. The chocolate should be poured on top of the cake.

Tropical Cheesy Fruit Salad

INGREDIENTS:

- 8 oz. mascarpone cheese
- 1/2 tsp. ground cinnamon
- 1 tsp. sugar
- 1/4 tsp. ground nutmeg
- 2 cups mandarin slices with juice. Spare 2 tbsp. of juice for later use
- 1/3 cup half-cut maraschino cherries with juice. Spare 2 tbsp. of juice.
- 1/2 cup un-drained crushed pineapple, canned
- 1 cup fresh/frozen mango chunks
- 1 cup tiny marshmallows
- 1/4 cup chopped fresh mint

Prep. time:
10 minutes

Cooking time:
35 minutes

Servings:
1 cup

DIRECTIONS:

1. Mascarpone, cinnamon, nutmeg, sugar, mandarin, and cherry juice should be whisked together for 1-2 minutes until smooth.

2. Mix the cherries, mandarin, pineapple, and mango pieces into the prepared mixture in a large mixing bowl.

3. Add marshmallows and mint on the top.

4. Serve it cold as a snack or dessert.

NUTRITION PER SERVING:

- Calories: 195 Cal
- Protein: 2 g
- Carbs: 20 g
- Fat: 13 g

Choco-Yogurt Muffins

INGREDIENTS:

- 1 can (15 oz.) drained and washed black beans
- 3 medium-sized eggs
- 1/3 cup cocoa powder, unsweetened
- 1/2 cup oats rolled
- 1/2 cup simple Greek yogurt
- 1/2 cup sugar
- 1 tsp. baking powder
- 1 tsp. minced orange zest
- 1 tsp. vanilla extract
- 1/2 cup less sweet chocolate chips or more for topping

NUTRITION PER SERVING:

- Calories: 141 Cal
- Protein: 5 g
- Carbs: 21 g
- Fat: 5 g

Prep. time:
15 minutes

Cooking time:
35 minutes

Servings:
12

DIRECTIONS:

1. Before you start cooking, preheat your oven to 350°F.

2. Coat the muffin molds with muffin liners or cooking spray.

3. In a blender, combine the eggs, beans, cocoa powder, and Greek yoghurt, as well as the rolled oats, sugar, orange zest, baking powder, and vanilla essence. In a blender, mix all of the ingredients to make a smooth batter.

4. Pour the batter into a medium mixing bowl and toss in the chocolate chunks.

5. In an equal layer, pour the batter into the muffin tins. Toss in some chocolate chips on top.

6. Cook for 25–30 minutes. Allow 5-10 minutes for chilling.

Fruit in The Clouds

INGREDIENTS:

- Fruit cocktail, 1 can drained
- Mandarin orange, 1 can drained
- Whipped cream, 8 oz frozen

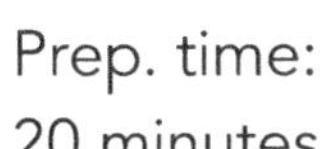

Prep. time:
20 minutes

Cooking time:
35 minutes

Servings:
4

DIRECTIONS:

1. Combine all ingredients in a mixing bowl.

2. Fill individual molds or an 8" × 8" container with the mixture. Freeze.

NUTRITION PER SERVING:

- Calories: 113 Cal
- Protein: 1 g
- Carbs: 23 g
- Fat: 3 g

Carrot Cake

INGREDIENTS:

- Granulated sugar, 1 cup
- Vegetable oil, 1/2 cup
- Eggs, 2
- Carrots, 1 1/2 cup, grated or shredded
- Vanilla extract, 1 tsp.
- All-purpose flour, 2 cups
- Nutmeg, 1/4 tsp.
- Baking soda, 2 tsp.
- Baking powder, 1 tsp.
- The ground cinnamon, 2 tsp.
- Ground cloves, 1/4 tsp.
- Pineapples, canned, 1 cup crushed

NUTRITION PER SERVING:

- Calories: 202 Cal
- Protein: 3 g
- Carbs: 30 g
- Fat: 8 g

Prep. time: 10 minutes

Cooking time: 15 minutes

Servings: 15

DIRECTIONS:

1. Preheat the oven to 375°F.
2. Combine the egg, oil, and sugar in a mixing bowl and whisk thoroughly.
3. Add the carrots and vanilla extract. Blend until a smooth consistency is achieved.
4. Combine the remaining ingredients in a large mixing bowl and stir thoroughly.
5. Pour the mixture into an oiled and floured 9" x 13" cake pan.
6. Preheat the oven to 350°F and bake for at least 30 minutes. Allow 10 minutes for cooling. Remove the pan from the heat.
7. Frosting on top or serve with whipped cream as a garnish (optional).

Old Fashioned Pound Cake

INGREDIENTS:

- Eggs, 6
- Butter, 2 cups
- Powdered sugar, 4 cups
- All-purpose flour, 3 1/2 cups, sifted
- Lemon rind, grated, 2 tbsps.
- Lemon extract, 1 tsp.

NUTRITION PER SERVING:

- Calories: 279 Cal
- Protein: 10 g
- Carbs: 34 g
- Fat: 12 g

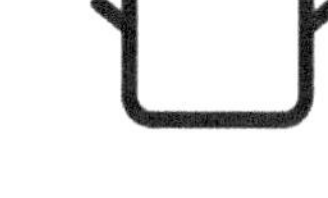

Prep. time:
25 minutes

Cooking time:
35 minutes

Servings:
24

DIRECTIONS:

1. Preheat oven to around 350°F. Using an electric mixer, cream butter on medium speed for around 3 minutes, or until creamy and light.

2. Slowly add the sugar and lemon peel and beat until completely combined.

3. One at a time, add the lemon extract and eggs, mixing thoroughly after each addition.

4. Slowly add the flour and fully combine.

5. Pour the mixture into a 10" Bundt pan or tube pan that has been oiled and floured.

6. Bake for nearly an hour and twenty minutes, or until a wooden pick inserted in the middle comes out clean.

7. Remove from the oven and set aside to cool.

Baked Egg Custard

  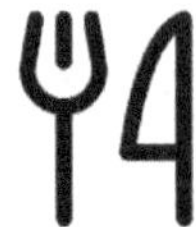

Prep. time:
10 minutes

Cooking time:
40 minutes

Servings:
4

INGREDIENTS:

- Eggs, 2, medium
- 2% milk, 1/4 cup
- Sugar, 3 tbsp.
- Vanilla, 1 tsp. (or lemon extract)
- Nutmeg, 1 tsp.

NUTRITION PER SERVING:

- Calories: 70 Cal
- Protein: 3 g
- Carbs: 9 g
- Fat: 3 g

DIRECTIONS:

1. Preheat the oven to 325°F.
2. Combine all ingredients in a mixing bowl and beat for one minute with an electric mixer until thoroughly combined.
3. Fill muffin tins or custard cups halfway with the mixture.
4. Put a pinch of nutmeg on each one.
5. Bake for around 20 to 30 minutes, or until a knife inserted in the center of the custard comes out clean.

Scarlet Frozen Fantasy

INGREDIENTS:

- Cranberry, 1 cup, juice cocktail

- Strawberries, fresh, whole, 1 cup, washed and hulled

- Lime juice, 2 tbsp., fresh

- Sugar, 1/4 cup

- Ice cubes, 8-9

- For garnish: strawberries

NUTRITION PER SERVING:

- Calories: 100 Cal

- Protein: 0 g

- Carbs: 24 g

- Fat: 0 g

Prep. time:
20 minutes

Cooking time:
35 minutes

Servings:
4

DIRECTIONS:

1. In a blender, combine the strawberries, cranberry juice, sugar, and lime juice. Blend well.

2. Adding ice cubes once more. Blend until completely smooth.

3. In cold glasses, serve. Add a strawberry as a finishing touch.

NOTES

7

Salads & Sause Recipes

White Wine-Herb Marinade with Tomatoes and

INGREDIENTS:

- 1 lb. chicken/fish/meat
- 1 cup dry white wine
- 1/2 cup lime juice
- 2 cloves garlic, minced
- 2 tbsp. fresh minced oregano
- 1 tbsp. fresh minced thyme
- 3 oz. crumbled feta cheese
- 2 chopped Roma tomatoes

NUTRITION PER SERVING:

- Calories: 76 Cal
- Protein: 2 g
- Carbs: 4 g
- Fat: 1 g

Prep. time:
5 minutes

Cooking time:
5 minutes

Servings:
6

DIRECTIONS:

1. Combine all items in a large mixing bowl or zip lock bag (excluding the protein).

2. Refrigerate the mixture for at least 30 minutes or up to a day in a zipped bag, turning or rotating periodically to ensure that the marinade is well distributed.

3. Take the protein meal out of the marinade and set it aside.

4. The protein is grilled on a low heat setting.

5. In a mixing dish, combine the cooked protein, tomatoes, and feta cheese.

Quick Pesto

INGREDIENTS:

- 40 fresh basil leaves
- 1 garlic clove
- 2 tbsp. walnuts
- 10 tbsp. shredded parmesan cheese
- 2/3 cup olive oil

NUTRITION PER SERVING:

- Calories: 334 Cal
- Protein: 4 g
- Carbs: 1 g
- Fat: 2 g

Prep. time:
5 minutes

Cooking time:
5 minutes

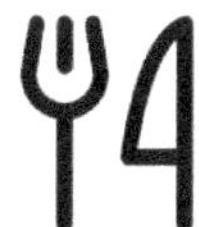

Servings:
6-8

DIRECTIONS:

1. All the ingredients, save the olive oil, should be finely blended in a blender.

2. Slowly pour in the oil while the engine is running to ensure that it is well blended.

Favorite American Blend

INGREDIENTS:

- 5 tsps. powdered onion
- 1/2 tsp. salt
- 1 tsp. thyme
- 1 tbsp. powdered garlic
- 1/2 tsp. white pepper
- 1 tbsp. paprika
- 1/2 tsp. celery seeds
- 1 tbsp. dry mustard

NUTRITION PER SERVING:

- Calories: 4 Cal
- Protein: < 1 g
- Carbs: < 1 g
- Fat: < 1 g

Prep. time:
10 minutes

Cooking time:
5 minutes

Servings:
32

DIRECTIONS:

1. Combine all the ingredients in an airtight container and thoroughly shake it.

Sour Cream Dip

INGREDIENTS:

- 8 oz. sour cream
- 1 tbsp.+1 tsp. Italian Medley Seasoning Blend
- 1 tsp. low-sodium Worcestershire
- 1/2 tsp. dried dill
- 1/2 tsp. paprika
- 1/2 tsp. onion powder

NUTRITION PER SERVING:

- Calories: 57 Cal
- Protein: < 1 g
- Carbs: 3 g
- Fat: 6 g

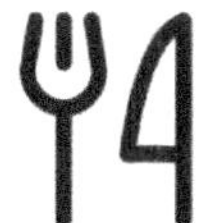

Prep. time:
10 minutes

Cooking time:
5 minutes

Servings:
8

DIRECTIONS:

1. Mix the sour cream and additional spices well with a fork.

2. Allow it to sit for at least one night.

French Style Vinaigrette

INGREDIENTS:

- 1 tsp. mustard
- 1 tsp. white vinegar
- 1 tsp. white wine vinegar
- 1/2 tsp. lime juice
- 3 tbsp. olive oil
- 1/4 tsp. minced garlic
- Pinch of Kosher salt
- 1/8 tsp. white pepper

NUTRITION PER SERVING:

- Calories: 91 Cal
- Protein: 8 g
- Carbs: < 1 g
- Fat: 10 g

Prep. time:
10 minutes

Cooking time:
5 minutes

Servings:
4

DIRECTIONS:

1. In a tightly sealed jar, combine all the ingredients.
2. Shake rapidly for 10 seconds, or until all ingredients are well mixed and the sauce looks creamy.

Asian Seasoning

INGREDIENTS:

- 2 tbsp. sesame seeds
- 2 tbsp. powdered onion
- 2 tbsp. ground star anise pods
- 2 tbsp. minced ginger
- 1 tsp. crushed allspice
- 1/2 tsp. cardamom
- 1/2 tsp. crushed cloves

NUTRITION PER SERVING:

- Calories: 10 Cal
- Protein: 0.3 g
- Carbs: 1 g
- Fat: 0 g

 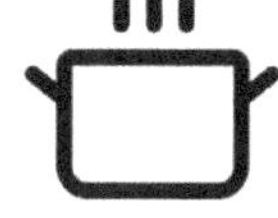

Prep. time:
10 minutes

Cooking time:
5 minutes

Servings:
1/2 cup

DIRECTIONS:

1. Combine all ingredients well.

2. Fill a small jar halfway with the spice mixture and seal it.

3. For up to five months, store it in a cool, dry location.

Creole Seasoning Mix

INGREDIENTS:

- 1 tbsp. paprika, sweet
- 1 tbsp. powdered garlic
- 2 tsps. powdered onion
- 2 tsps. dried oregano
- 1 tsp. cayenne pepper
- 1 tsp. crushed thyme
- 1 tsp. freshly crushed black pepper

NUTRITION PER SERVING:

- Calories: 7 Cal
- Protein: 1 g
- Carbs: 2 g
- Fat: 0.3 g

Prep. time:
5 minutes

Cooking time:
5 minutes

Servings:
1/4 cup

DIRECTIONS:

1. All the components should be well mixed together.

2. Half-fill a small jar with the spice mixture and seal it.

3. Store for up to six months in a cool, dry location.

Low-Sodium Mayonnaise

INGREDIENTS:

- 2 egg yolks
- 1 tsp. Dijon mustard
- 1 tsp. honey
- 2 tbsp. white vinegar
- 2 tbsp. fresh lime juice
- 2 cups olive oil

NUTRITION PER SERVING:

- Calories: 83 Cal
- Protein: 6 g
- Carbs: 38 g
- Fat: 9 g

 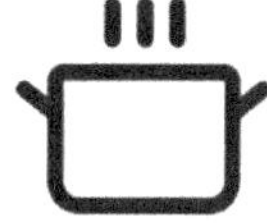

Prep. time:
10 minutes

Cooking time:
15 minutes

Servings:
3

DIRECTIONS:

1. Mix the mustard, egg yolks, honey, lemon juice, and vinegar in a mixing bowl.
2. Stir in the oil to get a smooth and thick mixture.
3. Refrigerate for two weeks in a tightly sealed glass jar.

Hot Curry Powder

INGREDIENTS:

- 1/4 cup crushed cumin
- 1/4 cup crushed coriander
- 3 tbsp. turmeric
- 2 tbsp. sweet paprika
- 2 tbsp. crushed mustard
- 1 tbsp. fennel powder
- 1/2 tsp. green chili powder
- 2 tsps. crushed cardamom
- 1 tsp. crushed cinnamon
- 1/2 tsp. crushed cloves

Prep. time:
10 minutes

Cooking time:
5 minutes

Servings:
1 ¼ cups

DIRECTIONS:

1. Combine all ingredients in a blender and mix until smooth.

2. Place the powder in a container that can be securely closed.

3. Store for up to six months in a cool, dry location.

NUTRITION PER SERVING:

- Calories: 19 Cal
- Protein: 1 g
- Carbs: 3 g
- Fat: 1 g

Herb Pesto

INGREDIENTS:

- 1 cup fresh basil leaves
- 1/2 cup fresh oregano leaves
- 1/2 cup fresh parsley leaves
- 2 garlic cloves
- 1/4 cup olive oil
- 2 tbsp. fresh lime juice

NUTRITION PER SERVING:

- Calories: 22 Cal
- Protein: 1 g
- Carbs: 9 g
- Fat: 2 g

 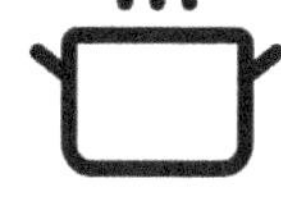

Prep. time:
5 minutes

Cooking time:
10 minutes

Servings:
1 ½ cups

DIRECTIONS:

1. 3 minutes in a blender, finely chop the garlic, basil, parsley, and oregano.

2. With olive oil and pesto, make a thick paste.

3. In a blender, squeeze the lemon juice and blend until smooth.

4. Refrigerate the pesto for up to 7 days in an airtight jar.

Dijon Vinaigrette

INGREDIENTS:

- 1 small-sized shallot
- 3 tbsp. lime juice
- 1 tbsp. red wine vinegar
- 1 tbsp. Dijon mustard
- 1/2 cup extra-virgin olive oil
- Pinch of freshly crushed black pepper

NUTRITION PER SERVING:

- Calories: 77 Cal
- Protein: 0 g
- Carbs: 1 g
- Fat: 8 g

Prep. time:
5 minutes

Cooking time:
5 minutes

Servings:
3/4 cups

DIRECTIONS:

1. Finely grate the shallot into a small bowl using a box grater.

2. Combine the red wine vinegar, lime juice, and mustard in a mixing bowl.

3. Drizzle in the olive oil gradually and season with pepper.

4. Place in an airtight container and keep refrigerated.

Homemade Barbeque Sauce

INGREDIENTS:

- 1 cup light brown sugar
- 2 cups fresh tomato sauce or 1 ½ cups Heinz ketchup
- 1/4 cup apple cider vinegar
- 1/2 cup water
- 2 tbsp. chili powder
- 2 tsps. paprika
- 1/4 tsp. black pepper
- 1/4 tsp. garlic powder
- 1/4 tsp. onion powder
- 1/4 tsp. garlic pepper
- 1/4 tsp. allspice
- 1 1/2 tbsp. organic crushed mustard
- 1 tsp. liquid smoke
- 1 tsp. Red-hot sauce
- 1 slash cayenne pepper

Prep. time: 10 minutes

Cooking time: 25 minutes

Servings: 4

DIRECTIONS:

1. Brown sugar, paprika, ketchup (or tomato sauce), water, vinegar, and chili powder in a saucepan for 2 minutes on low heat until smooth.

2. Combine the black pepper, powdered garlic, mustard, garlic powder, powdered onion, allspice, and liquid smoke in a large mixing bowl. Cook for a few minutes, or until the mixture is smooth.

3. Red-hot sauce and cayenne pepper should be combined (if using).

NUTRITION PER SERVING:

- Calories: 41 Cal
- Protein: < 1 g
- Carbs: 10 g
- Fat: < 1 g

Homemade Tomato Sauce

INGREDIENTS:

- 2 cups low sodium canned crushed tomatoes
- 1 small, diced onion
- 1/8 tsp. sea salt
- 4 tbsp. butter

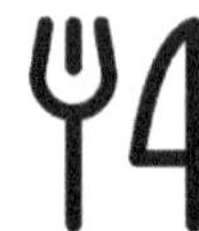

Prep. time:
20 minutes

Cooking time:
50 minutes

Servings:
6

NUTRITION PER SERVING:

- Calories: 85 Cal
- Protein: < 1 g
- Carbs: 4 g
- Fat: 8 g

DIRECTIONS:

1. Whisk together the butter, tomatoes, onion, and salt in a pan.

2. Over medium heat, bring to a boil.

3. Cook on low heat for 45 minutes or until it thickens, then serve hot.

Lemon Curry Chicken Salad

INGREDIENTS:

- 1/4 cup of vegetable oil
- 1/4 cup of frozen lemonade concentrate (thawed)
- 1/4 tsp. of ground ginger
- 1/4 tsp. of curry powder
- 1/8 tsp. of garlic powder
- 1 1/2 cups of chicken (cooked properly and diced)
- 1 1/2 cups of grapes (halved)
- 1/2 cup of celery (sliced)

NUTRITION PER SERVING:

- Calories: 276 Cal
- Protein: 15 g
- Carbs: 15 g
- Fat: 10 g

Prep. time:
5 minutes

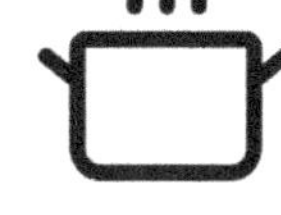

Cooking time:
20 minutes

Servings:
4

DIRECTIONS:

1. Combine the spices, oil, and lemonade concentrate in a mixing dish. Stir in the remaining ingredients gradually.

2. Allow approximately 1 hour for cooling.

Fall Harvest Orzo Salad

INGREDIENTS:

- 4 cups of cooked orzo and chilled (around 1 2/3 cups of dried orzo)
- 1 cup of dried cranberries
- 2 cups of fresh apples, diced
- 1/4 cup of extra-virgin olive oil
- 1/4 cup of fresh lemon juice
- 1/2 tsp. of freshly ground black pepper
- 2 tbsps. of fresh basil and chopped
- 1/2 cup of crumbled blue cheese
- 1/4 cup of blanched almonds (chopped)

NUTRITION PER SERVING:

- Calories: 289 Cal
- Protein: 6 g
- Carbs: 12 g
- Fat: 12 g

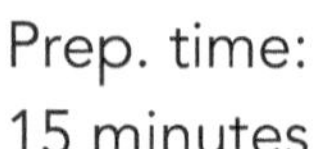  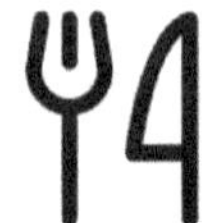

Prep. time:
15 minutes

Cooking time:
20 minutes

Servings:
8

DIRECTIONS:

1. Combine all the ingredients in a mixing bowl, except the almonds and blue cheese. Gently stir until everything is well combined.

2. To serve, transfer the mixture to a serving dish and top with almonds and blue cheese.

Mexican-Style Cucumber Salad

 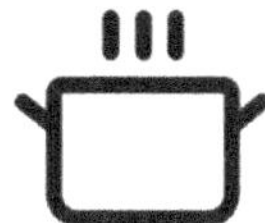

Prep. time:
15 minutes

Cooking time:
20 minutes

Servings:
4

INGREDIENTS:

- 1 large cucumber (sliced and peeled)
- 1/2 small size red onions (thinly sliced)
- Juice from 2 limes
- 1/2 tsp. of Mexican oregano

NUTRITION PER SERVING:

- Calories: 367 Cal
- Protein: 5 g
- Carbs: 29 g
- Fat: 0 g

DIRECTIONS:

1. Gently combine the red onion and cucumber in a mixing dish. Lime juice and oregano are added to the mix.

2. Cover and chill for 30 minutes to enable flavors to meld.

3. Chill or serve at room temperature. You may keep leftovers in the fridge for up to three days.

Mixed Green Leaf and Citrus Salad

INGREDIENTS:

- 4 cups of salad greens (mixed)
- 1/4 cup of pepitas
- Lemon juice of 1 lemon
- 2 tsps. of olive oil (extra virgin)
- Black pepper (freshly grounded) to taste
- 1 orange peeled (thinly sliced)
- 1/2 lemons peeled (thinly sliced)
- 4 tbsps. of (1/4 cup) dried cranberries
- 4 tbsps. (1/4 cup) of Kalamata olives (pitted)

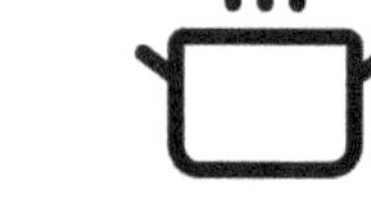

Prep. time:
5 minutes

Cooking time:
10 minutes

Servings:
4

DIRECTIONS:

1. Toss the olive oil, greens, pepitas, and lemon juice together in a mixing dish. Salt and pepper to taste.

2. In four separate bowls, divide the greens. 2 orange and lemon slices on each dish 1 tbsp. Cranberries and 1 tbsp. Kalamata olives are included in each dish.

NUTRITION PER SERVING:

- Calories: 134 Cal
- Protein: 3 g
- Carbs: 15 g
- Fat: 8 g

Summer Pasta Salad with White Wine

INGREDIENTS:

- 1 lb. of pasta noodles (such as farfalle, penne, rotini, or elbow)
- 1 large cucumber (sliced in half moons)
- 2 cups of arugula (coarsely chopped)
- 3 cloves of minced garlic
- 2 tbsp. of olive oil (extra virgin)
- 1 tbsp. of white wine vinegar
- Black pepper (freshly ground) to taste
- 1/4 cup of Parmesan cheese (grated)

NUTRITION PER SERVING:

- Calories: 238 Cal
- Protein: 9 g
- Carbs: 43 g
- Fat: 4 g

Prep. time: 15 minutes

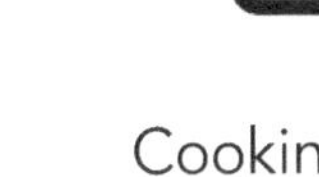
Cooking time: 25 minutes

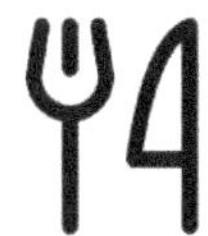
Servings: 8

DIRECTIONS:

1. Half-fill a dish with water and bring to a boil. Cook the pasta until it is al dente (firm but not mushy) (firm to the bite). To stop the cooking process, drain the pasta and rinse it with cold water.

2. Toss the cucumbers, noodles, garlic, and arugula together in a large mixing dish. Toss the salad with vinegar and olive oil after seasoning with pepper. Serve with a parmesan cheese sprinkle on top.

Bulgur Vegetable Salad

INGREDIENTS:

- 1 cup of cooked bulgur
- 1 cup of broccoli, chopped
- 1 cup of cauliflower, chopped
- 1 red bell pepper (finely diced)
- 1 scallion (green and white parts) chopped
- 2 tbsp. of basil leaves (fresh and chopped)
- Zest and juice of 1 lemon
- 1 tbsp. of olive oil
- Black pepper (freshly grounded) to taste

Prep. time: 10 minutes

Cooking time: 15 minutes

Servings: 5

DIRECTIONS:

1. Mix the cauliflower, bulgur, broccoli, bell pepper, basil, lemon zest, lemon juice, and olive oil in a large mixing bowl. Salt and pepper to taste.

2. Toss one more before serving.

NUTRITION PER SERVING:

- Calories: 106 Cal
- Protein: 3 g
- Carbs: 18 g
- Fat: 3 g

Cobb Salad

INGREDIENTS:

Dressing:

- 1/4 cup of olive oil
- 3 tbsp. of balsamic vinegar
- 1 tsp. of honey
- 1 tsp. of fresh thyme (chopped)
- Black pepper up to taste (freshly grounded)

Salad:

- 6 cups of baby greens (mixed)
- 1 cup of cherry tomatoes (cut in halved)
- 2 large eggs (hardboiled, peeled, smashed)
- 1 cup of cooked chicken breast (chopped)
- 1/4 ripe avocado pitted, peeled and diced

Prep. time:
5 minutes

Cooking time:
15 minutes

Servings:
6

DIRECTIONS:

To prepare the dressing:

1. In a mixing dish, combine the balsamic vinegar, oil, thyme, and honey. Salt and pepper to taste.

To prepare salad:

1. In a mixing bowl, combine the greens, eggs, cherry tomatoes, chicken, and avocado.

2. Place the salads on plates and pour the dressing over them.

NUTRITION PER SERVING:

- Calories: 172 Cal
- Protein: 11 g
- Carbs: 5 g
- Fat: 12 g

Peach Cucumber Salad

INGREDIENTS:

- 1 peach (peeled and cut in 1/2-inch cubes)
- 1 English cucumber (cut in 1/2-inch cubes)
- 1/2 cup of cherry tomatoes (halved)
- 1 scallion (green and white parts chopped)
- 1/2 cup of mint leaves (chopped)
- 1 tbsp. of lime juice (freshly squeezed)
- 4 cups of baby greens (mixed)
- Black pepper (freshly grounded) to taste

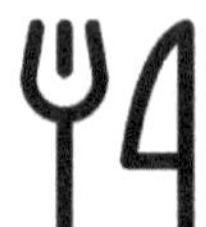

Prep. time:
5 minutes

Cooking time:
15 minutes

Servings:
4

DIRECTIONS:

1. Combine the peach, tomatoes, cucumber, scallion, lime juice, and mint in a mixing dish.

2. Top the leaves with the peach mixture in four separate bowls.

3. Season with pepper to taste and serve.

NUTRITION PER SERVING:

- Calories: 37 Cal
- Protein: 1 g
- Carbs: 1 g
- Fat: 0 g

Cranberry, Pepita, and Broccoli Salad

INGREDIENTS:

- 1/4 tsp. of smoked paprika
- 1/3 cup of mayonnaise
- 4 tsp. of apple cider vinegar
- 2 tbsp. of grated parmesan
- 1/3 cup of dried cranberries
- 2 scallions (chopped)
- 4 cups of 1 head broccoli (cut in small florets)
- 1/4 cup of unsalted and roasted pepitas
- Ground black pepper (fresh), to taste (optional)

NUTRITION PER SERVING:

- Calories: 147 Cal
- Protein: 3 g
- Carbs: 8 g
- Fat: 12 g

 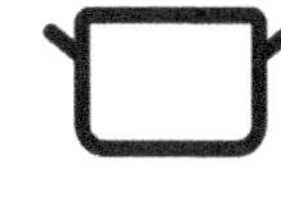

Prep. time: 10 minutes

Cooking time: 10 minutes

Servings: 6

DIRECTIONS:

1. Combine the parmesan, paprika, mayonnaise, and vinegar in a mixing dish.

2. In a large mixing bowl, combine the broccoli, cranberries, and scallions. Add the pepper and spices and mix well.

3. Place in the refrigerator until ready to serve. Before serving, scatter pepitas on top.

Kidney-Friendly Navy Bean Stew

INGREDIENTS:

- Navy Beans, Raw, mature seeds, 1 lb., Rinsed thoroughly
- Tomatoes, 2 can, packed in tomato juice (15 oz cans), no salt added
- Onion, 1, medium chopped
- Carrots, raw, 1cup grated
- Pepper, 2 tbsp.
- Seasoned 2.25 Oz
- Taste of Louisiana, 1/2 tbsp.
- Garlic, 3 cloves
- Chicken Bouillon, 2 cup, Sodium Free

NUTRITION PER SERVING:

- Calories: 264 Cal
- Protein: 17 g
- Carbs: 49 g
- Fat: 1.27 g

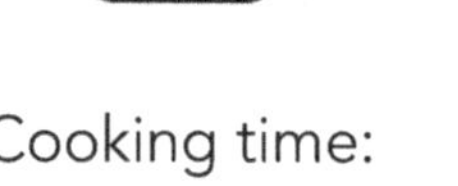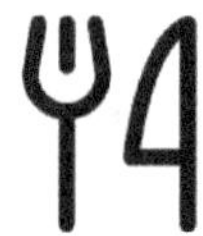

Prep. time: 10 minutes

Cooking time: 15 minutes

Servings: 6

DIRECTIONS:

1. 1 pound navy beans, cooked according to package instructions, should be immersed overnight.

2. Place the soaking water in a slow cooker.

3. Combine the onion, tomatoes, garlic, shredded carrots, Taste of the Louisiana Rub, black pepper, and chicken broth in a large mixing bowl.

4. Combine all ingredients and cook on lower heat for around 6-8 hours.

5. 1 cup should be poured into a serving dish and served right away.

6. If there is any leftover stew, it may be stored in the refrigerator for up to 3 days.

Chicken and White Bean Chili Stew

INGREDIENTS:

- Chicken breasts, boneless,1 pound, skinless
- Carrot, 3/4 cup
- Black pepper, 1 tsp.
- Celery, 3/4 cup
- Garlic, 4 cloves
- Onion, 3/4 cup
- White beans, 1 cup, canned
- Golden hominy, 15.5 oz. (1 can)
- Chicken broth, 4 cups, low-sodium
- Onions, white pearl, 6, whole
- Green chilies, diced, 4.5 oz canned
- Garlic powder, 2 tsp.
- Oregano, 1 tsp.
- Ground cumin, 2 tsp.
- Cayenne pepper, 1/4 tsp.
- Chili powder, 2 tsp.

NUTRITION PER SERVING:

- Calories: 213 Cal
- Protein: 19 g
- Carbs: 23 g
- Fat: 5 g

Prep. time: 20 minutes

Cooking time: 35 minutes

Servings: 8

DIRECTIONS:

1. Prepare the chicken by chopping it into tiny pieces. Place in the crock-pot and season with black pepper.

2. Celery, carrots, and onion should all be diced. Garlic should be finely chopped. Drain and rinse the beans and hominy to minimize sodium.

3. Combine the chopped onion, carrots, garlic, celery, hominy, beans, pearl onions, chicken broth, and green chilies in the crock-pot.

4. Garlic powder, chili powder, cumin, cayenne pepper, and oregano are all good additions.

5. Cook on low for 8 hours in the crock-pot with the lid closed.

Beef Casserole

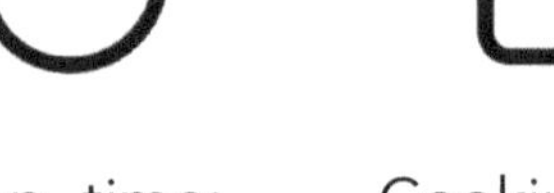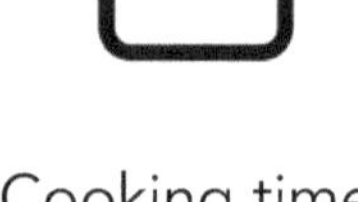

INGREDIENTS:

- Lean beef, 500g
- Chopped onion, 1 medium
- Carrots, 2, medium, peeled and sliced
- Water, 350 ml
- Salt, 1/4 tsp.
- Vegetable oil, 1 tbsp.
- White pepper, 1/4 tsp.
- Fresh parsley, 1 tbsp., chopped

NUTRITION PER SERVING:

- Calories: 304 Cal
- Protein: 23 g
- Carbs: 5 g
- Fat: 21 g

Prep. time:
15 minutes

Cooking time:
30 minutes

Servings:
4

DIRECTIONS:

1. In the vegetable oil, fry the chopped onion.
2. Add the meat and cook until it is brown.
3. Pour in the water and boil until the beef is nearly soft. Add the carrots and continue to cook until the meat and carrots are completely cooked.
4. Season with salt and pepper, then top with freshly cut parsley.

Chicken Stew

INGREDIENTS:

- Vegetable oil, 3 tbsp.
- Chicken breast, 2 pounds, cut into bite-size pieces
- Onions, sliced, 1 cup
- Green peppers, 3/4 cup
- Garlic, 2 cloves, minced
- All-purpose flour, 2 tbsp.
- Chicken broth, low-sodium, 2 10 1/2-oz cans
- Frozen carrots, 1 10-oz bag
- Dried basil, 1/4 tsp.
- Black pepper, 1/4 tsp.
- Sliced okra, frozen, 1 110-oz bag

NUTRITION PER SERVING:

- Calories: 142 Cal
- Protein: 10 g
- Carbs: 13 g
- Fat: 8 g

Prep. time:
10 minutes

Cooking time:
25 minutes

Servings:
4

DIRECTIONS:

1. Heat 2 tbsp. oil in a Dutch oven; add the chicken and cook over medium-high heat.

2. Remove the chicken and set it aside. 1 tbsp. extra virgin olive oil

3. Add the onion, garlic, and pepper and cook them together.

4. Cook, constantly stirring, for around 2 to 3 minutes after adding the flour.

5. Cook until the liquid and chicken begin to boil.

6. Cook for about 10 minutes, covered with carrots, black pepper, and basil. The gravy will thicken as it simmers.

7. Cook for another 5-10 minutes after adding the okra.

8. Serve over a bed of steaming white rice.

Chicken Cabbage Salad

INGREDIENTS:

Dressing:

- 1/2 cup of Mayonnaise (with low sodium)
- 2 tbsp. of apple cider vinegar
- 1 tsp. of sugar
- Black pepper (freshly grounded) to taste

Salad:

- 4 cups of cabbage (finely shredded)
- 1/4 cup of carrot (shredded)
- 2 scallions (green and white parts)
- 1 cup of chopped chicken breast (cooked)
- 2 tbsp. of fresh cilantro (chopped)
- 2 tbsp. of slivered almonds (toasted)

NUTRITION PER SERVING:

- Calories: 142 Cal
- Protein: 10 g
- Carbs: 8 g
- Fat: 13 g

Prep. time: 10 minutes

Cooking time: 20 minutes

Servings: 6

DIRECTIONS:

To prepare the dressing:

1. In a mixing dish, combine the vinegar, mayonnaise, and sugar mixture. Add a sprinkle of black pepper to taste.

To prepare salad:

1. Combine the carrots, cabbage, onions, cilantro, and chicken in a mixing dish.
2. Add salt and pepper to taste the salad.
3. Almonds may be added to the salad as a garnish.

Tabbouleh

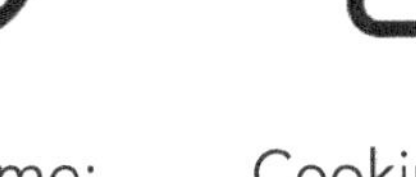

INGREDIENTS:

- 1 cup of medium bulgur (medium)
- 1 cup of cucumber (peeled and sliced)
- 1 cup of radish (thinly sliced)
- 4 scallions (sliced)
- 1 bunch of mint leaves (chopped)
- 2 lemons, juiced
- 1/2 cup of olive oil
- Freshly grounded pepper, to taste
- Kosher salt (optional), to taste

NUTRITION PER SERVING:

- Calories: 238 Cal
- Protein: 9 g
- Carbs: 43 g
- Fat: 4 g

Prep. time:
20 minutes

Cooking time:
30 minutes

Servings:
4

DIRECTIONS:

1. Half-fill a dish with hot tap water. In a large mixing bowl, combine bulgur and boiling water. Allow it to settle for at least 20-30 minutes, or until it has absorbed enough water. It should be avoided because of its messy appearance.

2. In a large mixing bowl, combine the chopped veggies and mint.

3. Remove any extra water from the bulgur by squeezing it.

4. Before serving, toss the salad with lemon juice. Mix everything with your hands or a big spoon after adding the olive oil. If required, season with salt and pepper to taste.

4. As a side dish, serve with fresh bread. Enjoy!

NOTES

7

Soups & Appetizers Recipes

Zucchini Sauté

INGREDIENTS:

- Fresh zucchini 4 medium-size, sliced
- Whole milk 1 cup
- Flour 1/2 cup
- Parmesan cheese 1/4 cup
- Fresh basil 1/2 tsp.
- Fresh thyme 1/2 tsp.
- Fresh tarragon 1/2 tsp.
- Vegetable oil 2 tbsps.
- To taste, pepper

Prep. time:
15 minutes

Cooking time:
20 minutes

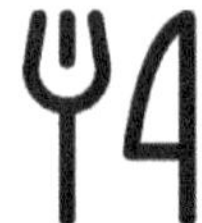

Servings:
4

DIRECTIONS:

1. Soak the zucchini in milk for a few minutes.
2. Add the herbs once the Parmesan cheese, flour, and pepper have been combined.
3. Heat the vegetable oil in a big skillet.
4. Zucchini should be dipped in a combination of cheese and herbs.
5. Serve right away.

NUTRITION PER SERVING:

- Calories: 121 Cal
- Protein: 6 g
- Carbs: 13 g
- Fat: 13 g

Spaghetti and Asparagus Carbonara

INGREDIENTS:

- Canola oil 2 tsps.
- Onions 1 cup fresh, diced
- Egg 1 large, beaten
- Heavy cream 1 cup
- 1/4 cup chicken stock (low-sodium)
- Spiral noodle pasta (about 1 1/2 cups)
- Fresh asparagus 2 cups, chopped
- Coarse black pepper 1 tsp.
- Fresh scallions 1/2 cup, chopped
- Bacon bits 3 tbsps.
- Parmesan cheese 3 tbsps.

NUTRITION PER SERVING:

- Calories: 304 Cal
- Protein: 9 g
- Carbs: 27 g
- Fat: 19 g

  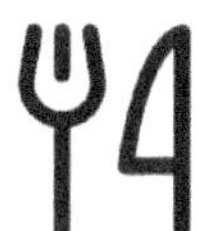

Prep. time: 15 minutes

Cooking time: 25 minutes

Servings: 6

DIRECTIONS:

1. In a large nonstick sauté pan, heat the oil over medium-high heat and cook the onions lightly browned.

2. In a medium mixing bowl, whisk together the egg and cream until completely mixed.

3. Reduce the heat to low and gradually whisk the cream mixture into the onions, stirring regularly with a wooden spoon until it thickens, approximately 4–6 minutes.

4. Stir for another 3–4 minutes, or until the asparagus, stock, pasta, and black pepper are completely warmed.

5. Place the carbonara in a serving dish after removing it from the heat. Bacon pieces, scallions, and cheese are served on top.

Grilled Multicolored Peppers and Onions

INGREDIENTS:

- Red onion 1 medium
- Vidalia onion 1 medium
- Yellow bell pepper 1
- Red bell pepper 1
- Green bell pepper 1
- Olive oil 1/3 cup
- Salt 1/4 tsp.
- Black pepper 3/4 tsp.

NUTRITION PER SERVING:

- Calories: 154 Cal
- Protein: 1 g
- Carbs: 11 g
- Fat: 13 g

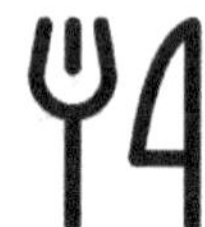

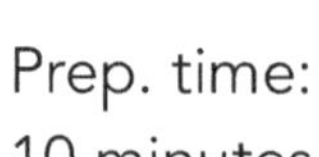

Prep. time:
10 minutes

Cooking time:
50 minutes

Servings:
2

DIRECTIONS:

1. Both onions should be quartered. Seeded bell peppers must be cut into 8 pieces.

2. Prepare a covered grill for direct cooking.

3. With a large mixing bowl, combine all ingredients and toss briskly to coat the vegetables in oil evenly.

5. Using metal skewers or a grill basket, arrange the vegetables. Grill for around 18 minutes, often turning to get even browning on both sides.

Green Pesto Pasta

INGREDIENTS:

- Whole wheat spaghetti 6 ounces, uncooked
- Basil leaves 2 cups
- Garlic 4 cloves
- 1/4 cup olive oil (extra virgin)
- Shredded parmesan cheese 2 tbsps.
- Black pepper 1/4 tsp.

NUTRITION PER SERVING:

- Calories: 303 Cal
- Protein: 8 g
- Carbs: 34 g
- Fat: 15 g

Prep. time: 12 minutes

Cooking time: 40 minutes

Servings: 6

DIRECTIONS:

1. Bring a saucepan of water to a boil, then cook the pasta as directed on the box, omitting the salt. Drain.

2. To chop the garlic, basil leaves, and Parmesan cheese, pulse them in a food processor. Drizzle the olive oil slowly into the basil mixture and blend until smooth, scraping down the sides of the mixer as needed.

3. Add pepper to taste.

4. Mix the spaghetti with the basil pesto sauce just before serving to coat it properly.

Red Wine Vinaigrette Asparagus

INGREDIENTS:

- Garlic 1 clove
- Fresh asparagus 2 pounds
- Olive oil 1 tbsp.
- Vinaigrette dressing (red wine) 1/4 cup
- Black pepper 1/2 tsp.

NUTRITION PER SERVING:

- Calories: 58 Cal
- Protein: 2 g
- Carbs: 6 g
- Fat: 3 g

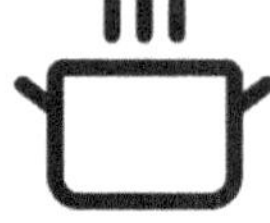

Prep. time:
10 minutes

Cooking time:
20 minutes

Servings:
4

DIRECTIONS:

1. Asparagus should be cut into 2" pieces, and garlic should be minced.
2. Heat the oil in a pan and sauté the garlic for 1 minute
3. Toss in the asparagus and mix well.
4. Pepper and red wine vinaigrette dressing are used to season the salad.
5. Heat for an additional minute after adding the other ingredients.
6. Serve immediately after removing the pan from the heat.

Creamy Grape

INGREDIENTS:

- Seedless grapes 3 pounds
- 8 ounces cream cheese, low-fat
- Sour cream 8 ounces
- Sugar 1/2 cup
- Vanilla extract 2 tsps.

NUTRITION PER SERVING:

- Calories: 168 Cal
- Protein: 2 g
- Carbs: 22 g
- Fat: 8 g

Prep. time:
20 minutes

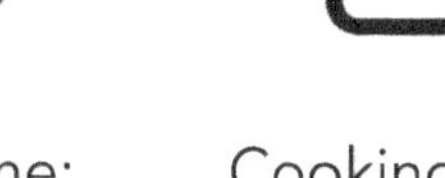

Cooking time:
30 minutes

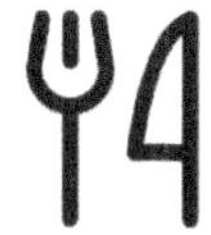

Servings:
3

DIRECTIONS:

1. To soften the cream cheese, place it in the refrigerator.
2. Grapes must be sliced in half vertically.
3. Combine sour cream, sugar, softened cream cheese, and vanilla extract in a medium mixing dish.
4. The grapes should be folded into the mixture.
5. Chill the dish before serving.

Almost Mashed Potatoes

INGREDIENTS:

- Cauliflower 6 cups
- Cream cheese 4 ounces
- Garlic 1 tsp.
- Black pepper 1/2 tsp.

  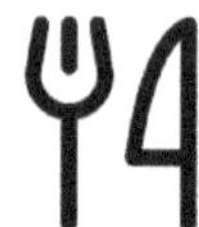

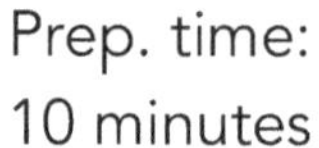

Prep. time:
10 minutes

Cooking time:
25 minutes

Servings:
1

NUTRITION PER SERVING:

- Calories: 94 Cal
- Protein: 3 g
- Carbs: 6 g
- Fat: 7 g

DIRECTIONS:

1. Cauliflower should be washed and chopped into pieces.

2. Place the cauliflower pieces in a microwave-safe dish, cover, and cook high for 8 to 10 minutes, or until soft.

3. Any extra liquid from cooked cauliflower should be drained.

4. Place your heated cauliflower in a blender and mix until smooth.

5. In a mixing bowl, combine the garlic, cream cheese, and pepper. Use a blender to mix the items.

6. After removing the mixture from the mixer, serve immediately.

Beet and Cucumber Salad

INGREDIENTS:

- Cucumber 1
- Canned sliced beets 15 ounces
- Balsamic vinegar 4 tsps.
- Canola oil 2 tsps.
- Gorgonzola cheese 2 tbsps.

NUTRITION PER SERVING:

- Calories: 174 Cal
- Protein: 1 g
- Carbs: 13 g
- Fat: 2 g

Prep. time:
10 minutes

Cooking time:
15 minutes

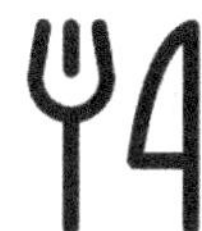

Servings:
1

DIRECTIONS:

1. Thinly slice the cucumber.
2. Arrange sliced beets on a serving platter.
3. On top of the beet slices, place cucumber slices.
4. Drizzle with olive oil and balsamic vinegar before serving.
5. Top with Gorgonzola cheese.

Cauliflower in Mustard Sauce

INGREDIENTS:

- Dijon mustard 2 tsp.
- Honey 1 tsp.
- White wine vinegar 2 tsp.
- Olive oil 1 tbsp.
- Black pepper, a dash
- Cauliflower flowerets 2 cups

NUTRITION PER SERVING:

- Calories: 51 Cal
- Protein: 1 g
- Carbs: 5 g
- Fat: 4 g

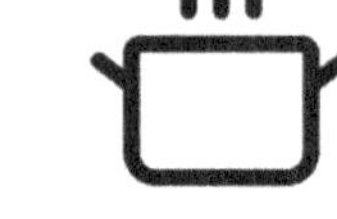

Prep. time:
15 minutes

Cooking time:
30 minutes

Servings:
2

DIRECTIONS:

1. After whisking together, the mustard and honey, add the vinegar and olive oil.

2. To taste, add a sprinkle of black pepper.

3. In a saucepan of boiling water, cook the cauliflower until it is tender.

4. Drain the water completely.

5. Once the cauliflower has been rinsed, toss it with the dressing.

6. Allow 30-45 minutes for chilling before serving.

Cool Coconut Marshmallow Salad

 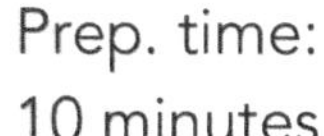  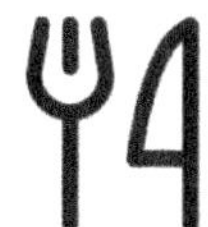

Prep. time:
10 minutes

Cooking time:
25 minutes

Servings:
8

INGREDIENTS:

- Fruit flavored marshmallows 1 package
- Dried coconut 1 cup
- Fruit cocktail 1 can
- Sour cream 2 cups

NUTRITION PER SERVING:

- Calories: 317 Cal
- Protein: 3 g
- Carbs: 40 g
- Fat: 18 g

DIRECTIONS:

1. Combine all the ingredients in a mixing bowl.

2. Pour into a glass bowl to serve.

3. If you want a creamy salad, chill it for an hour before serving. If you want the salad to be more molded, refrigerate it overnight.

Fresh Fruit Compote

INGREDIENTS:

- Strawberries 1/2 cup
- Blackberries 1/2 cup
- Blueberries 1/2 cup
- Peaches 1/2 cup
- Red raspberries 1/4 cup
- Orange juice 1/2 cup
- Apple 1, sliced
- Banana 1, sliced

NUTRITION PER SERVING:

- Calories: 44 Cal
- Protein: 0.5 g
- Carbs: 11 g
- Fat: 0.2 g

Prep. time:	Cooking time:	Servings:
12 minutes	25 minutes	4

DIRECTIONS:

1. Half-fill a large container with orange juice.
2. In a mixing dish, combine all the ingredients.
3. Toss gently.
4. Allow the frozen fruit to thaw at room temperature for 4 hours.

Italian Eggplant Salad

 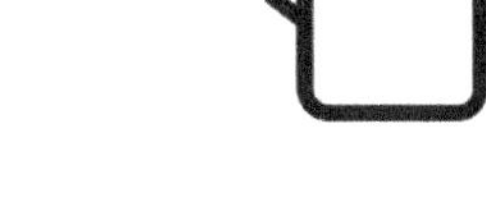 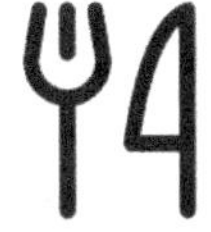

Prep. time:
15 minutes

Cooking time:
25 minutes

Servings:
4

INGREDIENTS:

- Eggplant, 3 cups
- Small onion, 1 chopped
- White wine vinegar 2 tbsp.
- Garlic 1 clove, chopped
- Oregano 1/2 tsp.
- Black pepper 1/4 tsp.
- Tomato 1 medium, chopped
- Olive oil 3 tbsp.

NUTRITION PER SERVING:

- Calories: 69 Cal
- Protein: 1 g
- Carbs: 6 g
- Fat: 5 g

DIRECTIONS:

1. Add the eggplant to the boiling water in a saucepan.
2. Bring the water to a boil, then remove from the heat.
3. Cook for 10 minutes, covered, or until tender; drain.
4. Combine the eggplant and onion in a glass dish.
5. In a mixing dish, combine the garlic, vinegar, and pepper.
6. In a large mixing bowl, combine the eggplant and onion with the sauce.
7. Add the oil just before serving.

Low Salt Macaroni and Cheese

INGREDIENTS:

- Noodles, 2 cups
- Boiling water 3 cups
- Cheddar cheese 1/2 cup, grated
- Margarine 1 tsp.
- Dried Mustard 1/4 tsp.

NUTRITION PER SERVING:

- Calories: 163 Cal
- Protein: 6 g
- Carbs: 20 g
- Fat: 7 g

Prep. time:
10 minutes

Cooking time:
20 minutes

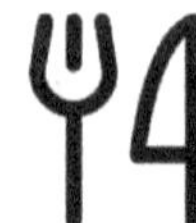

Servings:
4

DIRECTIONS:

1. Bring a pot of water to a boil, then add the noodles and simmer until soft, about 5-7 minutes.

2. Drain all the water.

3. While still hot, sprinkle with cheese and mix with butter and mustard. (For added crunch, bake for 10 - 15 minutes at 350°F or until golden brown on top.)

Cucumber Cups Stuffed with Buffalo Chicken

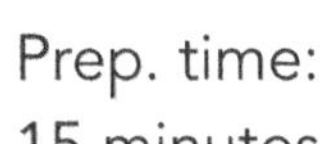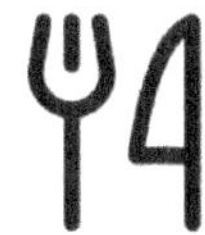

Prep. time:
15 minutes

Cooking time:
20 minutes

Servings:
8

INGREDIENTS:

- Black pepper 1/2 tsp.
- Smoked paprika 1 tsp.
- Italian seasoning 1/2 tsp.
- Cayenne pepper 1 tsp.
- Hot sauce 2 tbsps.
- Kraft mayonnaise 1/2 cup
- Blue cheese crumbs 1/2 cup
- Lemon juice 2 tbsps.
- Fresh garlic 1 tbsp., chopped
- Fresh chives 2 tbsps., chopped
- Chicken breast 3 cups, diced
- Cucumbers 2 large seedless
- Fresh parsley 1/4 cup, chopped

DIRECTIONS:

1. Combine all the ingredients in a medium mixing bowl, except the chicken and cucumbers.

2. In a large mixing bowl, toss in the chicken until it is uniformly coated. Refrigerate for around 30 minutes before serving.

3. Remove the cucumber slices from the fridge and pour 1–2 tsps. of mayonnaise into each one. Garnish with chopped parsley before serving.

NUTRITION PER SERVING:

- Calories: 132 Cal
- Protein: 2.3 g
- Carbs: 12 g
- Fat: 2 g

Curried Carrot Soup

INGREDIENTS:

- Avocado oil 4 tablespoons
- Onion, diced 1 medium
- Baby carrots 1 1/2 lbs.
- Fresh ginger 1 1/2-inch
- Curry powder 1 1/2 tablespoons
- Pepper flakes 1/2 teaspoon
- Vegetable broth low sodium 3 cups
- Coconut milk 1 can
- Sea salt 1/4 teaspoon
- Black pepper 1/4 teaspoon

NUTRITION PER SERVING:

- Calories: 256 Cal
- Protein: 3 g
- Carbs: 16 g
- Fat: 25 g

Prep. time:
10 minutes

Cooking time:
30 minutes

Servings:
6

DIRECTIONS:

1. Add some avocado oil to a saucepan and warm on medium heat. Once the oil is hot, add the chopped onion and simmer for 5-10 minutes, until tender and aromatic.
2. Continue to simmer for a further 5 minutes, or unless ginger is aromatic, before adding any baby carrots and chopped ginger back into the pan.
3. Once you've added your curry powder and pepper flakes, continue toasting for 30-60 seconds while mixing to release the aroma. Don't let the spices get too hot or they may burn.
4. Toss in some vegetable broth and coconut milk after the spices have begun to smell good. Then reduce the heat, cover, and allow the carrots simmer for around 15-20 minutes until they are tender.
5. Once your carrots are tender, gently mix the soup with the immersion blender till it is smooth and creamy. Alternatively, allow the soup to cool somewhat before blending in batches in a strong blender. Add salt and pepper to your liking and mix well.
6. Add lemon juice and coconut milk to your soup just before serving it.

Herbed Cream Cheese Toasts

INGREDIENTS:

- Melba toast rounds 20
- Garlic 1 clove, sliced
- Cream cheese 1 cup
- Mixed herbs 1/4 cup
- Onion 2 tbsp.
- Black pepper 1/2 tsp.
- Water 2 tbsp.

NUTRITION PER SERVING:

- Calories: 79 Cal
- Protein: 2.6 g
- Carbs: 10 g
- Fat: 2.3 g

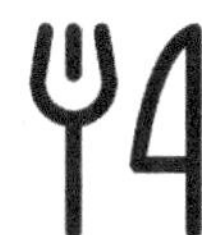

Prep. time:
25 minutes

Cooking time:
35 minutes

Servings:
10

DIRECTIONS:

1. In a medium mixing bowl, combine herbs, cream cheese, shallot, pepper, and water using a handheld mixer.

2. With the cut edge of the garlic slice, rub it on the bread.

3. Cream cheese should be served on toasted bread.

Blueberry Brie

INGREDIENTS:

- Brie Cheese 1 wheel, 2.2 pounds

- Blueberry pie filling 1, 16 oz.

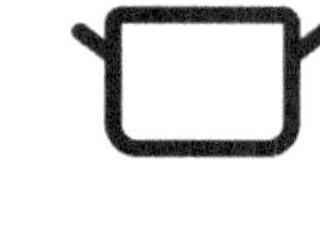

Prep. time:
10 minutes

Cooking time:
15 minutes

Servings:
4

NUTRITION PER SERVING:

- Calories: 118 Cal

- Protein: 6.5 g

- Carbs: 3.8 g

- Fat: 8.6 g

DIRECTIONS:

1. Preheat your oven to 350°F.

2. Using one side of a Brie, remove the rind. Maintain the rind's border and bottom.

3. Brie should be placed in a baking dish with blueberry pie filling on top.

4. Preheat oven to 350°F and bake for around 10 to 15 minutes, or until heated.

5. Allow it to cool slightly before serving with crackers or baguette slices from France.

Baked Pita Chips

INGREDIENTS:

- Pita rounds 3
- Olive oil 3 tbsp.
- Chili powder

 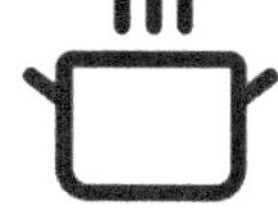

Prep. time: 14 minutes

Cooking time: 40 minutes

Servings: 3

NUTRITION PER SERVING:

- Calories: 137 Cal
- Protein: 2.5 g
- Carbs: 15.4 g
- Fat: 7 g

DIRECTIONS:

1. Cut pitas into two rounds using kitchen scissors. Eight wedges should be cut from each pita. Season pita slices with chili powder and drizzle with olive oil. Preheat the oven to 350°F and bake for 15 minutes, or until crisp.

Quick 'n' Easy Cheese Dip

INGREDIENTS:

- Cottage cheese 1-1/2 cups
- Sour cream 1 cup
- Green onions 3
- Tabasco hot sauce 2 tsps.
- Dill weed 1 tsp.
- Garlic powder 1/2 tsp.
- Crumbled blue cheese 1/3 cup

NUTRITION PER SERVING:

- Calories: 78 Cal
- Protein: 4 g
- Carbs: 3 g
- Fat: 5 g

Prep. time:
15 minutes

Cooking time:
45 minutes

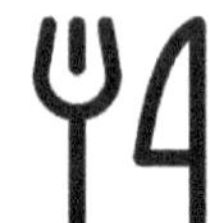

Servings:
3

DIRECTIONS:

1. Combine cottage cheese, green onions, sour cream, spicy sauce, and spices in a food processor and pulse until smooth.

2. After adding the blue cheese, mix for a few more seconds.

3. Garnish with chopped green onion if desired.

Festive Pineapple Cheese Ball

INGREDIENTS:

- Cream cheese 24 ounces
- Crushed pineapple 20 ounces
- Green bell pepper 1/2 cup
- Garlic powder 1/2 tsp.

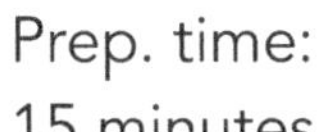

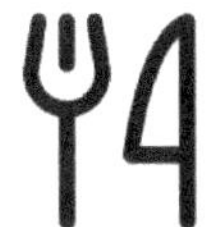

Prep. time:
15 minutes

Cooking time:
35 minutes

Servings:
2

DIRECTIONS:

1. In a large mixing bowl, soften the cream cheese.

2. The pineapple should be completely drained. Bell peppers should be cut into tiny bits.

3. To blend the components, combine them in a mixing bowl and thoroughly whisk them together.

4. Assemble the components into a ball. Refrigerate overnight after wrapping with wax paper.

NUTRITION PER SERVING:

- Calories: 95 Cal
- Protein: 2 g
- Carbs: 4 g
- Fat: 10 g

Sugar and Spice Popcorn

INGREDIENTS:

- 8 cups popcorn, air-popped
- Unsalted butter 2 tbsps.
- Sugar 2 tbsps.
- Cinnamon 1/2 tsp.
- Nutmeg 1/4 tsp.

NUTRITION PER SERVING:

- Calories: 120 Cal
- Protein: 2 g
- Carbs: 12 g
- Fat: 7 g

 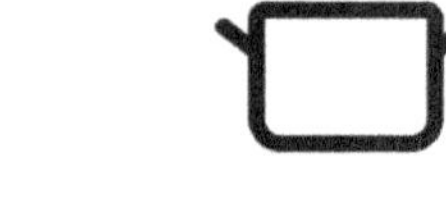 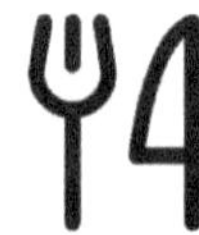

Prep. time:
15 minutes

Cooking time:
10 minutes

Servings:
2

DIRECTIONS:

1. In a saucepan, heat the butter, cinnamon, sugar, and nutmeg until the butter has melted, and the sugar has dissolved. If preferred, heat the mixture in a microwave-safe dish. Keep an eye on the butter to make sure it doesn't burn.

2. Toss the spiced butter mixture with the popped popcorn to incorporate.

3. Serve immediately.

Shrimp Spread with Crackers

INGREDIENTS:

- Light cream cheese 1/4 cup
- Shelled shrimp 2-1/2 ounces
- Ketchup, 1 tbsp.
- Tabasco hot sauce 1/4 tsp.
- Worcestershire sauce 1 tsp.
- Herb seasoning blend 1/2 tsp.
- Matzo cracker miniatures 24
- Parsley 1 tbsp.

NUTRITION PER SERVING:

- Calories: 57 Cal
- Protein: 3 g
- Carbs: 7 g
- Fat: 1 g

 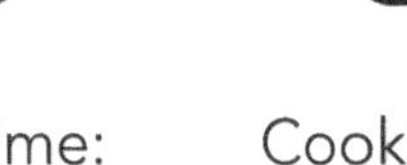 

Prep. time:
10 minutes

Cooking time:
12 minutes

Servings:
3

DIRECTIONS:

1. Refrigerate the cream cheese to soften it.
2. Mince the shrimp and combine it with the cream cheese in a mixing dish.
3. Toss in the herb seasoning, ketchup, Tabasco sauce, Worcestershire sauce, and ketchup.
4. Spread 1 spoonful of the spread on each cracker. Garnish with parsley, if desired.

Snack Mix

INGREDIENTS:

- Rice cereal squares 1 cup
- Corn cereal squares 1 cup
- 1 cup pretzel twists, unsalted
- 3 cups popcorn, unsalted
- 1/3 cup margarine
- Garlic powder 1/2 tsp.
- Onion Powder 1/2 tsp.
- Parmesan cheese 1 tbsp.

NUTRITION PER SERVING:

- Calories: 180 Cal
- Protein: 2 g
- Carbs: 19 g
- Fat: 11 g

Prep. time:
10 minutes

Cooking time:
12 minutes

Servings:
8

DIRECTIONS:

1. Preheat your oven around 350°F

2. Pretzels, cereals, and popcorn should all be combined in a big mixing bowl.

3. Toss the garlic and onion powders into the melted margarine. To coat the cereal, toss it in the sauce. At this stage, you may add the parmesan cheese.

4. Preheat the oven to 350°F and bake for around 7 to 10 minutes.

5. Before serving, let it cool completely.

6. Keep in a container with a tight lid.

NOTES

Abbreviations

lb. Pound

c. Cup

tbsp. Tablespoon

gal. Gallon

qt. Quart

min. Minute

oz. Ounce

°F Degree Fahrenheit

T. Tablespoon

pt. Pint

tsp. Teaspoon

hr. Hour

Equivalents

1 cup = 16 tbsps.

3/4 cup = 6 fluid ounces

2 quarts = 4 pints

1/2 pound = 8 ounces

8 tbsps. = 1/2 cup

1/2 tbsp. = 1 ½ tsp.

1/4 cup = 4 tbsps.

1 pound = 2 cups

5 gallons = 20 quarts

12 fluid ounces = 1.5 cups

3 ½ hours = 210 minutes

1/8 cup = 1 fluid ounces

40 ounces = 2.5 pounds

3 tsps. = 1 tbsp.

16 tbsps. = 1 cup

1 pound = 16 ounces